POSTTRAUMATIC PLAY IN CHILDREN

Also from Eliana Gil

Cultural Issues in Play Therapy
Edited by Eliana Gil and Athena A. Drewes

Essentials of Play Therapy with Abused Children (DVD)
Eliana Gil

Helping Abused and Traumatized Children:
Integrating Directive and Nondirective Approaches
Eliana Gil

Play in Family Therapy, Second Edition
Eliana Gil

Play Therapy for Severe Psychological Trauma (DVD)
Eliana Gil

Termination Challenges in Child Psychotherapy
Eliana Gil and David A. Crenshaw

The Healing Power of Play: Working with Abused Children
Eliana Gil

Treating Abused Adolescents
Eliana Gil

Working with Children to Heal Interpersonal Trauma:
The Power of Play
Edited by Eliana Gil

Working with Children with Sexual Behavior Problems
Eliana Gil and Jennifer A. Shaw

Posttraumatic Play in Children

What Clinicians Need to Know

Eliana Gil

THE GUILFORD PRESS
New York   London

The author has checked with sources believed to be reliable in her efforts to provide
information that is complete and generally in accord with the standards of practice
that are accepted at the time of publication. However, in view of the possibility of
human error or changes in behavioral, mental health, or medical sciences, neither the
author, nor the editor and publisher, nor any other party who has been involved in
the preparation or publication of this work warrants that the information contained
herein is in every respect accurate or complete, and they are not responsible for any
errors or omissions or the results obtained from the use of such information. Readers
are encouraged to confirm the information contained in this book with other sources.

Library of Congress Cataloging-in-Publication Data

Names: Gil, Eliana, author.
Title: Posttraumatic play in children : what clinicians need to know / Eliana Gil.
Description: New York : The Guilford Press, [2017] | Includes bibliographical
   references and index.
Identifiers: LCCN 2016044537 | ISBN 9781462528820 (paperback) |
ISBN 9781462528837 (hardcover)
Subjects: | MESH: Play Therapy—methods | Child Abuse—therapy | Child
Classification: LCC RJ505.P6 | NLM WS 350.4 | DDC 618.92/891653—dc23
LC record available at https://lccn.loc.gov/2016044537

To Myriam Goldin and Jennifer Shaw, my best friends and my inspiration in everything I do. I thank you for your unconditional support, your incredible loyalty, and our shared vision. You are my playmates, my business partners, and the most ethical and talented of colleagues. I rejoice that you are in my life.

About the Author

Eliana Gil, PhD, is founding partner of the Gil Institute for Trauma Recovery and Education, a private group practice in Fairfax, Virginia. She is also Director of Starbright Training Institute for Child and Family Play Therapy. Dr. Gil has worked in the field of child abuse prevention and treatment since 1973. A licensed marriage, family, and child counselor; an approved marriage and family therapy supervisor; a registered art therapist; and a registered play therapy supervisor, she is a former president of the Association for Play Therapy, which honored her with its Lifetime Achievement Award. She is the author of *The Healing Power of Play, Helping Abused and Traumatized Children,* and *Play in Family Therapy, Second Edition,* among many other publications. Originally from Guayaquil, Ecuador, Dr. Gil is bilingual and bicultural.

Preface

*R*ecent decades have seen profound advances in research into working with traumatized children (Ford & Courtois, 2013; Lanktree & Briere, 2017). Breakthroughs in neuroscience over the past 15 years have been particularly fruitful for practitioners (Perry, 2001; Perry & Szalavitz, 2006; Perry & Dobson, 2013). Consensus has been reached on the domains typically affected by trauma, specifically the areas of attachment, emotional and behavioral regulation, biology, dissociation, cognitive functioning, and identity. In addition, the National Child Traumatic Stress Network (NCTSN; *www.nctsn. org*) cites specific critical aspects of trauma-informed therapy: (1) safety, (2) self-regulation, (3) self-reflective information processing, (4) integration of traumatic experiences, (5) relational health, and (6) enhancement of positive affect. What remains in question are the specific interventions that might advance treatment goals and assist children's recovery process.

Diverse treatment approaches continue to vie for legitimacy, especially because some approaches (like play therapy) are more difficult to operationalize and research than others. Only a small percentage of the clinical community has the funding or the academic setting necessary to conduct research. Several evidence-based therapies are recommended, especially trauma-focused cognitive-behavioral therapy (TFCBT; Cohen, Mannarino, & Deblinger, 2006). Yet like every other treatment approach, TFCBT cannot be effective with every client, especially those who have expressive language deficits, are very young and have linguistic or cognitive limitations, or have firmly entrenched avoidance. There is professional agreement that exposure techniques are necessary components of trauma-informed therapy. However, dissociation is particularly resistant to exposure techniques. More and more, the literature on traumatized children reports the necessity to incorporate play, art, or other expressive therapies in the assessment and treatment of young children, whether directive or nondirective techniques are used.

So while we recognize that several evidence-based programs have empirical support for positive treatment outcomes, other approaches are widely used and clinically useful, though not yet empirically supported.

My early work with posttraumatic play focused on its progression and the variables suggesting whether or not the play meets its intended goal. When posttraumatic play fails to provide children with mastery and to reduce anxiety, I suggest that it has become stagnant and potentially problematic—stagnant posttraumatic play may retraumatize children and make things worse for them rather than better. I first published a list of factors for clinical vigilance in 1998 (Gil, 1998). As a trainer who has provided educational programs on this topic to thousands of mental health professionals, I have found that many clinicians struggle with how to assess when posttraumatic play is helpful and when it is not, and how to intervene when necessary. Even when the play does not provide relief, it can supply valuable assessment information about children's posttraumatic stress.

Diagnosis of traumatized children who don't meet the full criteria for posttraumatic stress disorder (PTSD) as established in DSM-5 has always been challenging. The Zero to Three categorizations create opportunities to view posttraumatic responses in a different light, in a way that is perhaps more consistent with children's developmental changes. However, research has shown that most children have several of the symptoms associated with posttraumatic stress, and recent efforts have been directed at designing assessment instruments that are developmentally sensitive, particularly with very young children (Stover & Berkowitz, 2005).

In fact, based on current criteria for PTSD, it can be concluded that children manifest unique repetitive play that can signal the re-experiencing of trauma. Posttraumatic play clearly manifests literal elements of the traumatic event and, more importantly, can provide a self-reparative mechanism that is internally driven. Early findings on childhood trauma suggest that posttraumatic play is done in secret. However, I believe that children will exhibit posttraumatic play in the clinical setting when they view it as a warm and inviting setting, when there is a willing and receptive witness to the play, and when clinical interventions are permissive and allow the play to unfold until more directive interventions might be necessary.

I am convinced that we clinicians don't always know better. You can remain as informed as possible, prepare yourself continuously, and then, as Carl Jung (1928) said, "learn your theories as well as you can, but put them aside when you touch the miracle of the living soul. Not theories, but your own creative individuality alone must decide" (p. 361). The privilege of helping others comes with great responsibility and requires constant reevaluation of what we are doing. I believe that while we all tend to develop a certain level of comfort with our theories and approaches, we should always remain open to being surprised and inspired by the children with whom we work. They know best how to contribute to their own well-being. In other words, children can and will lead the way. We clinicians should therefore follow their lead unless it becomes necessary to supplement what they are doing in other important ways. This is the crux of *Posttraumatic Play in Children*.

It is my hope that this book supplements and amplifies the descriptive, anecdotal, and empirically based discussion of posttraumatic play to date and that it will be a useful resource for both play therapists and nonplay therapists who work with traumatized children.

GRATITUDE

In this book I am eager to share what I have learned over the years on this amazingly pivotal topic. My professional career with clients is suspended at the moment with what may or may not be a permanent semi-retirement. It is with great pleasure that I now look back and organize my thoughts on a topic that is so important to me. Perhaps this will be my last book. If so, and if it reaches its intended audience and contributes to clinical consideration and creative, flexible thinking, I will be immensely pleased.

I express my sincere gratitude to a small group of individuals who have sparked and shaped my interest, inspired my work, and helped me strive for excellence in my professional role with children and their families. My thanks to Spencer Eth, Robert Pynoos, Lenore Terr, Judith Herman, Katherine Nader, Lucy Berliner, Janine Shelby, Charles Schaefer, Bruce Perry, John Briere, Cheryl Lanktree, and Phyllis Booth. A special note of thanks to Bessel van der Kolk for spearheading a movement to introduce a new diagnostic category—developmental trauma disorder—into the DSM system and for always advocating for child and adult survivors of trauma. This diagnostic category is unequivocally the best way to evaluate the impact of trauma on young children and will hopefully make its way into a future version of the DSM.

Finally, what I learned from Garry Landreth, though not specific to trauma per se, provided an important context in all the work I did with children. It allowed me to prioritize *relationship* when working with children (and their families). My gratitude is endless.

Contents

— *Part I* —

Understanding
Posttraumatic Play

1

Introduction to Posttraumatic Play in Children and Youth

*T*his book is written for treatment professionals. The goal is simple: to inform or strengthen clinical understanding of how posttraumatic play is an essential component of children's trauma recovery. Rather than presenting posttraumatic play as a method that originates with the clinician, in this volume, it is viewed as the creative product of the child—a remarkable personal reparative strategy that usually emerges in the context of unconditional acceptance, patience, careful observation, and purposeful, individually tailored responses.

Although attention has consistently been given to how to identify posttraumatic play in children, less attention has been paid to clinical issues important in the emergence and facilitation of posttraumatic play in therapeutic settings. Thus, my focus in this book is on exploring how clinicians might better understand posttraumatic play and provide informed and responsible interventions to optimize positive treatment outcomes.

This book focuses primarily on Type II traumas, those that are understood to be complex trauma cases, chronic and disturbing in their unrelenting stress effects on children. They include multiple types of abuse and multiple perpetrators. Also included are beginning research on the impact of Type I traumas (such as hurricanes, terrorism, and earthquakes) and some examples of children with Type I traumas.

I view posttraumatic play as a type of play that needs clinical recognition and facilitation, but it can be categorized more accurately as a form of child resilience—an effort to process and manage traumatic memories and as such it is definitely a phase of trauma-informed treatment. Dynamic posttraumatic play that achieves its intent of mastery greatly adds to the recovery process, but it is not a singular solution. Rather, it occurs in the context of a larger treatment picture in which other issues such as attachment, self-regulation, cognitive and perceptual shifts, self-esteem, and identification of resources will need to be addressed.

Within that larger treatment picture, posttraumatic play can be seen as gradual exposure, or systematic desensitization; this type of behavior therapy has been shown effective in helping clients overcome phobias and other anxiety disorders. Gradual exposure consists of exposing the client to the situation that he or she fears. This exposure can decrease intense emotions to the feared situation, to the point that anxiety subsides and the client feels more in charge.

BENEFITS OF PLAY

To fully appreciate the value and benefits of posttraumatic play, it is important to consider the benefits of play in general. Play has been used in child therapy since the early 20th century as a means for children to communicate and make sense of their experiences (Bratton, Ray, Rhine, & Jones, 2005). Schaefer and Drewes (2010) have noted that several therapeutic (or curative) factors in play give children opportunities for self-expression, access to the unconscious, abreaction, learning, stress inoculation, counterconditioning of negative affect, catharsis, positive affect, relationship enhancement, and others. In their more recent volume (2013), Schaefer and Drewes expand on their earlier work, discussing the empirical evidence that supports each therapeutic factor in play therapy, the techniques that can advance each factor, and the reasoning that supports why play therapy can contribute to the child's growth and development through health-promoting capacities. Marans, Mayes, and Colonna (1993) note that play helps young children rework difficult experiences and makes their actions predictable and their behavior less anxiety-provoking. They also claim that play may allow children to give a less negative meaning to their sometimes chaotic experiences. The noted psychologist Erik Erikson (1802–1994) asserted that playing out traumas is the most natural self-therapeutic process childhood offers and that children will repeat everything in their play that has made a great impression on them (Erikson, 1950). While playing out traumas, Erikson observed, children abreact the strength of the trauma, making it manageable and less intense. These abreactive experiences offered through play can lead such children to develop feelings of mastery. Clearly, play and therapy have great potential to help traumatized children, especially since they will need "a variety of expressive means and projective techniques" given their often limited ability to directly reflect and verbally report about their thoughts and feelings (Nader & Pynoos, 1991).

A LOOK AHEAD

In the rest of this chapter, I review the effects that trauma can have on children, discuss the nature and distinguishing characteristics of posttraumatic play, and then review clinical approaches to posttraumatic play. Chapter 2 goes into more detail on the types of posttraumatic play, the forms it can take, and the phases it often undergoes. There are two main types of posttraumatic play. When it is positive and therapeutic, I call it *dynamic* posttraumatic play. When it becomes stuck, posing the danger of retraumatizing the child, I call this type *toxic* posttraumatic play. Chapter 3 describes how to assess posttraumatic play, how to differentiate toxic from dynamic play, and when and how to intervene when play is toxic. Chapter 4 details how posttraumatic play can manifest itself in natural settings such as at school or hospital and in the therapy office. Chapter 5 provides an overview of the larger treatment context in which posttraumatic play has a pivotal role. In addition to individual therapy, treatment may include parallel work with parents, conjoint narrative sharing, psychoeducation, attachment-based work, and reunification services. Chapters 6 through 13 offer detailed clinical illustrations of posttraumatic play, profiling a range of children who have experienced both Type II and Type I traumas. Finally, the case presented in Chapter

14 illustrates the larger treatment context, specifically, parallel work with a parent and conjoint narrative sharing, which becomes possible following the child's posttraumatic play.

THE EFFECTS OF TRAUMA ON CHILDREN

Over the past three decades, many clinicians have championed the plight of traumatized children and their recovery and have led the way in providing necessary information for those working with this vulnerable population (Eth & Pynoos, 1984, 1985; Saywitz, Mannarino, Berliner, & Cohen, 2000). We have many accounts of children responding to traumas in unique ways that are expressive (e.g., Goodman & Fahnestock, 2002). There are also relevant case studies on how children respond to catastrophes (see, e.g., Cohen, Chazan, Lerner, & Maimon, 2010; Thabet, Karim, & Vostanis, 2006; Saylor, Swenson, & Powell, 1992).

Spencer Eth and Robert Pynoos (Eth & Pynoos, 1985) have been exceptionally prolific and single-minded in studying trauma effects on children. They asserted that children experience and express traumatic stress differently than adults and so need a different response (Pynoos & Nader, 1989, 1990, 1993; Pynoos, Nader, & March, 1991; Pynoos & Eth, 1985; Eth & Pynoos, 1984, 1985). Eth and Pynoos's pioneering work caused a shift in thinking, which is reflected in DSM-III-R's list of symptoms of posttraumatic stress disorder (PTSD) specific to children, such as "nightmares of monsters, of rescuing others by superhuman powers, and of threats to self or others . . . tending to relive the trauma in their play without realizing they are doing it . . . regressive behaviors (encopresis, enuresis), and somatic complaints (headaches stomachaches)" (Schaefer, 1994, p. 297).

Stover and Berkowitz (2005) stated that "posttraumatic stress phenomena influence a number of developmental processes. . . . Prominent personality changes. . . . Regressive behaviors and a marked change in attitude toward the future" (p. 707). Kilpatrick and Williams (1998) note that "frequently found patterns of symptoms of PTSD in children include regression to earlier developmental stages, nightmares that they may generalize into less specific monster nightmares, post-traumatic play in which children re-enact the trauma, daydreaming, and difficulties concentrating frequently associated with academic under-achievement" (p. 319). Mental health professionals generally agree that adverse events in childhood can contribute to the emergence of a broad range of psychological, social, and emotional problems later on. At the same time, a number of mediating factors have been identified in traumatized children, including "the child's age and gender, locus of control, coping style (active versus palliative), presence or absence of self-blame, the child's perception of the threat, and the mother's level of emotional well-being" (Gibbs, 1989) (Kilpatrick & Williams, 1998, p. 320). Marvasti (1994) cautioned that traumatic meaning may differ depending on the cultural lens used to assess its importance and to determine appropriate adaptive mechanisms. I have worked with cultures in which women and children are massively marginalized and abused routinely. These victims often develop a "move forward, don't look back" approach that serves them well, given the predictability and normalcy of abuse in their lives. Some mothers thus support their children in forgetting, moving forward, and trying to defuse the power of the abuse over their lives.

Cohen et al. (2010) cite Salmon and Bryant (2002), who stated that children are particularly vulnerable to overwhelming stressors: "immaturities in emotional regulation, social cognition, information processing, language, and memory act together to impact upon available coping responses in young children when faced with traumatic events. These immaturities particularly impact upon integration of the traumatic memory into the self-schema of the child" (p. 161).

In spite of advances in identifying posttraumatic stress signs in children, assessment remains challenging: "The inherent difficulty in assessing a complex psychological disorder with children who may not have the ability to understand or verbalize their own internal experiences is clear" (Stover & Berkowitz, 2005, p. 714). It is worth noting that efforts to introduce a more appropriate diagnostic category—developmental trauma disorder—into DSM-5 that might more fully capture the range of posttraumatic concerns in children were not successful in spite of massive support for this addition by trauma specialists (van der Kolk, 2005).

Lenore Terr, a San Francisco psychiatrist, asserted that, in childhood, "psychic trauma leads to a number of mental changes that eventually account for some adult character problems, certain kinds of psychotic thinking, considerable violence, much dissociation, extremes of passivity, self-mutilative episodes, and a variety of anxiety disturbances" (1991, p. 11). Terr provided a comprehensive definition of trauma: "I will define childhood trauma as the mental result of one sudden, external blow or a series of blows, rendering the young person temporarily helpless and breaking past ordinary coping and defensive operations" (p.11).

Terr also differentiated between conditions that were sudden and unexpected and those conditions marked by children's "prolonged and sickening anticipation," but she affirmed that all childhood traumas originated externally. Forecasting contemporary interest in biology, Terr predicted that "childhood trauma may be accompanied by as yet unknown biological changes that are stimulated by external events" (1991, p. 11). With the advent of brain scan technology, scientists and neurobiologists have provided a wealth of information on brain changes during trauma, which now inform and guide clinical interventions (Levine & van der Kolk, 2014, 2015; Perry & Szalavitz, 2006; Perry, 2001). Nader and Pynoos (1991) cite growing evidence "that neurobiological alterations may occur when the child's adaptive responses are overwhelmed by the traumatic experience, particularly when it is in the form of maltreatment" (p. 116).

Terr (1991) has a singular interest in childhood traumas, noting that in addition to the more common characteristics of childhood trauma ("thought suppression, sleep problems, developmental regressions, fears of the mundane, deliberate avoidances, panic, irritability, and hypervigilance," p. 12), other features prevail. She specifies that four other factors are critical: "strongly visualized or otherwise repeatedly perceived memories, repetitive behaviors, trauma-specific fears, and changed attitudes about people, aspects of life, and the future" (p. 12). Other researchers have posited four categories that appear unique to children's stress response (Fenichel, 1994): re-experiencing of the traumatic event (usually through posttraumatic play or nightmares and flashbacks); numbing of responsiveness; increased arousal; and new symptoms not present before the traumatic event. One of Terr's most intriguing statements is that children (especially those under 5) do not always have repetitive posttraumatic dreams—the repetitive dream is what she considers a *hallmark of trauma*. I have often wondered if posttraumatic play doesn't serve the same purpose as dreaming, that is, to access unconscious material during a trance-like state. Posttraumatic play often has the quality of "awake sleeping" (compartmentalizing) that allows for images, sensations, feelings, and cognitions to come to the surface for processing.

Terr described two types of childhood trauma: Type I, which includes incidents such as kidnapping, witnessing murder, dog attack, and car crash; and Type II, which is more chronic and tends to have an interpersonal component. She rarely documented Type II traumas in her early studies; the exception involved two victims of satanic, ritual abuse for which there might have been an interpersonal aspect. I believe that the posttraumatic play of children with Type I and II traumas may be different: Type II posttraumatic play may last longer, be less receptive to clinical interpretation, and need more time to reach fruition. Terr (cited in Schaefer, 1994) noted that Type I traumas "do not appear to exhibit the massive denial, psychic numbing, dissociation, depersonalization, rage, or personality disorders that characterize the Type II traumas" (p. 298). More comparative studies are needed that distinguish posttraumatic play of children with Type I and II traumas.

DEFINING POSTTRAUMATIC PLAY

Lenore Terr coined the term *posttraumatic play* and has provided most of the foundational information we presently have for the types and characteristics of posttraumatic play. She studied the play behaviors of 26 children from two separate traumatic incidents. As a result of her clinical observations, she identified a unique type of play which she called *posttraumatic play*. Terr has done seminal, rigorous work on the impact of trauma on child development. She has also maintained a long-term interest in children's play following trauma (Terr, 1981, 1991), including documentation of the characteristics of posttraumatic play, based in particular on a longitudinal study of children kidnapped in Chowchilla, California (Terr, 1992). She found that unlike other play in children, posttraumatic play was repetitive, rigid, literal, devoid of pleasure, and, most importantly, failed to produce the usual gains, such as decreasing children's anxiety. What became most apparent in her studies was the driven and relentless quality of the play.

Terr's information was based on a fairly small sample of children (total $N = 26$) who underwent catastrophic trauma and then played out their experiences. This study has prompted further study designed to verify Terr's findings. Findling, Bratton, and Henson (2006), for example, found support for the idea that "the play behaviors of traumatized children differ from the play behaviors of children with no known history of trauma and that the differences concur with Terr's construct of post-traumatic play" (p. 26). Other professional efforts are underway to design or improve upon available measures for evaluating traumatic experiences and their impact on children, including the emergence of symptoms of PTSD (Stover & Berkowitz, 2005). All in all, it is clear that children's play must be taken into account and remains relevant in any work with young, traumatized children (Stover & Berkowitz, p. 707).

Terr's Characteristics of Posttraumatic Play

Terr notes that posttraumatic play, in contrast to generic play, is devoid of the child's experience of having fun and fails to relieve his or her anxiety. She further defined posttraumatic play by listing the following 11 characteristics (discussed in more detail in Terr in 1981):

1. *Compulsive repetition of play,* which Terr (1981) believes will not stop until children "are told by parents or teachers to stop, until they are sent away, or until they reach an emotional understanding of the connection of their play to the original psychic trauma" (p. 744). When discussing treatment of childhood trauma, Terr often limits her guidance to a psychoanalytic use of interpretation that links the play to actual events. She states strongly that therapeutic interpretation allows children to finally reach the insight needed to relieve the anxiety that she believes drives the play.

2. *An unconscious link between the play and the trauma.* Terr believes that the primary clinical function is to provide therapeutic interpretations, which in many of the cases she describes, appear to have positive and immediate impact. It might be important to note

here that Terr believes that most children are not likely to demonstrate posttraumatic play in a clinical setting (a very different finding from my own).

3. *The play is literal.* Terr describes the play as "less elaborate" than generic play and goes on to talk about simple defenses in the play.

4. *Failure of play to relieve anxiety.* This particular factor receives a great deal of Terr's attention. She obtains her reports of the anxiety prior to her work with children, believing that once interpretations are given, the play stops. In some of the cases of Type II traumas I have handled, the children seem to present posttraumatic play only after establishing relational safety in the therapy relationship. It may be the unconditional accepting witness by the clinician which allows the child to become increasingly capable of tolerating the play as it unfolds in the clinical setting. I have also had different experiences with interpretation, finding that children resist being told what they think or feel or having the actual events taken out of the more distant role of pretend play.

5. *Wide age range.* Terr documents a wide range of "players," noting that posttraumatic play "extends to a wider age range than does ordinary play" (p. 748).

6. *The play may start at various times posttrauma.* Terr notes varying lag times prior to the start of posttraumatic play, ranging from fairly immediate to months later.

7. *The play can pull in nontraumatized children.* Terr also observes that this anxious play can "pull in" nontraumatized youngsters. This makes sense given that children commonly want to engage others in their play. In my experience, many traumatized children don't interact with the clinician, which sets the play apart from most nontraumatized children who like to interact and role-play with others.

8. *A contagious quality.* Terr also documents the contagious quality of this play, which has the potential to impact others.

9. *Some posttraumatic play can become dangerous.* Play involving behavioral reenactments of the trauma can place the child or others at risk. Thus, clinicians are well advised to evaluate the type and

extent of the play and with whom and where it surfaces, if it occurs outside the clinical setting.

10. *Use of doodling, talking, and audio duplication* as modes of repeated play.

11. *The possibility of tracing posttraumatic play to an earlier trauma.*

Terr emphasizes that posttraumatic play differs from ordinary play in that ordinary play "carries with it a 'cure,' an opportunity to fully identify with a well-meaning aggressor (parent, doctor or teacher) or an opportunity to turn the tables and spank a doll or give shots to a younger sibling. No one is hurt, abreaction occurs, and the child is able to diminish the anxiety after a few play episodes" (p. 755). She notes that when children attempt to use posttraumatic play to relieve anxiety, they fail. Further, children cannot identify with those who have hurt them and feel threatening to them. In the Chowchilla kidnapping, she states that none of the children were able to play the part of "Jack," the bus driver who had terrorized them; they could not identify with his level of cruelty. The full "pretend identification" is thus not possible; there is a "failure of distancing" (p. 756). Terr's basic assertion is that children believe that (their formerly reliable) play activities might help them address their underlying issue, but when trauma occurs, play fails to provide the relief they seek.

My views on the topic of anxiety relief differ from Terr's because, as stated above, the bulk of my experience has been in a clinical setting. My primary approach has always been integrative, which allows child-centered play to proceed uninterrupted so that I can assess whether play repetition eventually allows for the introduction of new elements. Something new and different might emerge, and relief might occur. I assume that initially posttraumatic play will be constricted, but with time it will evolve into greater free play, leading to more ample risk-taking through various forms of expression and ultimately to physical, sensory, creative, or expressive release. (These differences are discussed in subsequent chapters.)

My view of posttraumatic play is most consistent with Schaefer's belief that play, in general, has many "curative factors." Among these factors is the possibility of abreactive work, which is greatly facilitated through repetition and which "seems to weaken the negative affect associated with the trauma and strengthens a sense of mastery of the event in the child" (Schaefer, 1994, p. 301). I call such therapeutic play *dynamic* posttraumatic play. Schaefer also cites "retraumatizing play," which I describe as *toxic* play, a type of play that needs more direct intervention so that positive outcomes can occur. Schaefer states that "post-trauma play has a greater chance of achieving mastery for children when they 1) feel in control of the outcome of the play; 2) play out a satisfactory ending to the play; 3) feel free to express and release negative affect; and 4) exhibit a cognitive reappraisal of the event" (p. 308). My clinical perspective and experience line up completely with this view: play has significant healing components for traumatized children! Stover and Berkowitz (2005) noted the value of play for traumatized children in plain words: "Simply stated, the younger a child is the less they are able to understand a potentially traumatic event (PTE) and adequately report how their emotions are tied to that event" (p. 708).

CLINICAL APPROACHES TO POSTTRAUMATIC PLAY

Freud first discussed the concept of compulsive repetition early in his work; he thought the repetition could signal the presence of a conflict that was deeply embedded in the client's unconscious mind and thus could not be properly resolved. However, he believed that every repetition in play weakens the negative affect associated with the trauma, thus giving children the feeling that they are more in control and less overwhelmed (Freud, 1914/1958). This concept has inspired several treatment approaches, including release therapy (Levy, 1938), active play therapy (Solomon, 1938), and mastery play therapy. Schaefer (1994), in a discussion of mastery play therapy, concluded that "child therapists are combining abreaction, cognitive reappraisal, a supportive relationship, and crisis intervention principles in their play therapy approach to psychic trauma" (p. 308).

Shelby and Felix (2005) wrote an important update on the topic of posttraumatic play therapy and reviewed the advantages and disadvantages of directive and nondirective approaches with traumatized children. They noted that, "in general, the literature supports the use of directive, trauma-focused therapy over nondirective, support-oriented techniques to reduce most child trauma symptoms," with the exception of one study that found no significant therapy outcome differences when working with children with sexual behavior problems (p. 82). However, traumatized children tend to have a prominent difficulty with avoidance and will resist many directive approaches. Thus, Shelby and Felix (2005) point to "a number of intuitive advantages" of nondirective work based on anecdotal evidence showing that it can feel more "gentle" and satisfying to child clients. They also maintain that both approaches can be helpful, but the integration of the two allows clinicians to tailor therapy interventions to the specific children who seek their help. Dripchak (2007) describes an Eriksonian approach with posttraumatic play that "uses both directive and nondirective strategies" and requires "neither insight nor interpretations of the unconscious for change" (p. 127). She goes on to say that "its focus is on the present perceptions of the child and on future acceptance and solutions," using the child's potential and resources.

Shelby and Felix propose an evidence-informed treatment framework that they call posttraumatic play therapy; their therapy expands on the standard practice of including a mixture of cognitive-behavioral approaches, supportive, and psychodynamic psychotherapy. The basic components of this perspective are parental involvement, developmentally sensitive interventions, and specific techniques. Shelby and Felix provide a practical set of guidelines for trauma-sensitive therapists to use. A particularly useful portion of their work is a list of common trauma symptoms and the empirically based interventions that respond best to specific concerns. This innovative assessment-driven therapy approach has also been advocated by Lanktree and Briere (2017) in their recent book on working with young children.

Shelby describes a powerful technique that she used when she worked with 56 young trauma survivors following Hurricane Andrew, a Type I trauma (1999). This technique is called *experiential mastery* (Shelby, 1997) and is congruent with the theory of mastery play therapy. Schaefer (1994, p. 315) discusses this type of play therapy, stating that "the mastery play therapy approach should be comprehensive and utilize such strategies such as crisis intervention, abreaction, affective expression, exposure techniques, cognitive reappraisal, and social support." These factors are components of most contemporary treatment programs with traumatized children to one degree or another.

Shelby's experiential mastery technique appears to facilitate crisis intervention, abreaction, and affective expression. It is considered an exposure technique and is likely influenced by the important art interview originally described by Pynoos and Eth (1986). Shelby asked children to draw pictures of whatever frightens them the most and express their feelings to the drawings, and she then instructed them to do whatever they wished to their drawings. In this way, children are asked to externalize their feelings, express their emotions, and take some kind of action that engenders their sense of mastery. Interestingly, several art-focused trauma interventions currently enjoy popularity (Chapman, 2014a; Malchiodi, 2012; Tinnin & Gantt, 2013). Neuroscience has greatly expanded the ways therapists can view art and other expressive therapies in the assessment and treatment of childhood trauma (Malchiodi, 2003).

Finally, Shelby and Felix (2005) caution clinicians to recognize and accept that any treatment recommendations relating to methods of treating traumatized children are "based on a markedly incomplete and evolving knowledge base" (p. 98). They conclude that "it falls to us as trauma treatment developers to humbly acknowledge that our most valuable teachers are our clients themselves" (p. 98).

My approach, trauma-focused integrated play therapy (TFIPT; Gil, 2012), is integrative; Shelby and Felix (2005) refer to it as a "mastery therapy" and Saunders, Berliner, and Hanson (2003) as a "promising practice." It is heavily influenced by Judith Herman's work and her three phases of treatment. The TFIPT model includes the application of child-centered play therapy as an introductory approach with all clients, and it is designed to allow children to access reparative strategies by (1) following their pace in treatment; (2) offering the therapy relationship as the context for their work; and (3) facilitating, valuing, encouraging, or helping children process posttraumatic play. Within the TFIPT model, integration is highly prized, so the polarized discussion of whether or not to use directive or nondirective strategies is a moot issue, one that is decided by the child's receptivity, learning style, defensive strategies, self-pacing, as well as clinical judgment. The initial agenda is set by children and it is altered only when it does not satisfy its positive intent. TFIPT relies on evidence- and practice-informed methodologies. In this approach, posttraumatic play is highly valued as one of the change agents for traumatized children.

CONCLUSION

Posttraumatic play can be understood as a natural reparative strategy exhibited by many traumatized children. This type of play mimics the behavioral intervention of gradual exposure. During posttraumatic play, children externalize painful or frightening thoughts and feelings through symbol, metaphor, story, or play. Sometimes literal objects provide avenues for children to share their experiences. Other times children use symbolic play to maintain the safe enough distance they require to play out their concerns. Posttraumatic play appears to be a pivotal feature of children's overall recovery process and usually occurs within the context of a permissive and safe therapeutic environment.

It is a given that children abused by parents, caretakers, and other trusted individuals will struggle with additional challenges that present themselves when they have been abused by those they might depend on and love. My clinical experience suggests that children work out very diversified issues when they have experienced complex trauma—multiple abusers, chaotic homes, chronic abuse, all of which affect normative child development. By definition, complex trauma requires that children be able and willing to trust in the therapist and the therapy process, be receptive to an unconditionally accepting witness, and be capable of accessing natural reparative resources, namely, posttraumatic play.

The next chapter explores the characteristics of posttraumatic play in greater depth, including its positive and negative aspects, the forms it can take, and the phases it can often undergo.

2

Types, Forms, and Phases
of Posttraumatic Play

Maria Fernanda's uncle was killed in a Level 7 earthquake when she was 5 years old. She witnessed his entrapment from a distance as he disappeared in the rubble, wood, and wires. The child looked away as her uncle was buried, and she cried for months, asking where he was and whether he would return. Her mother would remind her that her uncle was now buried in the cemetery and took her to place flowers. Her mother told me that Maria Fernanda would dig small holes in the dirt, placing dead bugs that she collected during the week. Every Thursday afternoon (coincidentally, the day of the earthquake), she dug small holes, buried dead bugs, and said prayers at their graves. Eventually, she brought live bugs to the holes and watched intently as they climbed out. She repeated this play over and over, until she stopped. Slowly, her mother said the child returned to her previous happy state, although any intensely hot weather terrified her.

Maria Fernanda's mother did not interrupt or inhibit her child's behavior. She knew intuitively that this type of play was serving a purpose for her daughter. For Maria Fernanda, it appears that the play she utilized (as well as possibly the passage of time) was helpful in allowing her to return to the sense of security she had enjoyed—and taken for granted—prior to the earthquake. But not all children are able to resolve their traumas in this manner, and many of them don't enjoy the optimal nurturing of concerned parents who make efforts to reassure their children after a sudden, unexpected catastrophic trauma (Type I traumas).

Maria Fernanda's mother seemed to have a ready appreciation for the reparative nature of her child's posttraumatic play, but many parents can minimize or ignore the impact of traumatic events. Some parents may become very concerned when they notice the presence of non-normative play following a trauma. They may try to stop or discourage their children's posttraumatic play, preferring that they "forget" negative or difficult events and move on. Such parents often hold on to the hope that if children forget traumatic events, then all difficult feelings such as anxiety or fear will also cease. Therefore, it becomes critical to educate parents and professionals alike about the desirability and potential benefits of spontaneous posttraumatic play, as well as some of the warning signs and dangers when this play may not be producing positive outcomes.

Elsewhere these two types of posttraumatic play have been simply called positive and negative, with the positive allowing children to "modify the negative components of the trauma" and the negative showing that "the repetitive play is unsuccessful in relieving anxiety and fails to help the child attain resolution or acceptance" (Marvasti, 1994, p. 126). I call the first type *dynamic* posttraumatic play and the second *toxic* to highlight the differences and the ongoing need to observe all aspects of the play's evolution. These distinctions will then guide clinical decisions on whether to allow or actively intervene in children's posttraumatic play.

DYNAMIC POSTTRAUMATIC PLAY: THE POSITIVE INTENT

Dynamic posttraumatic play is designed to allow children to externalize their memories and to advance from a passive stance to a more active one in which they decide *when* and *what* to remember. Too often, children with traumatic histories use defensive strategies such as denial, suppression, or repression. This compartmentalizing defensive strategy spares children from immediate pain, but it has long-term consequences. When traumatic memories are unresolved, there is a greater chance that children will act out or develop symptomatic behavior that may be less than adaptive. Their self-esteem may suffer, their relationships may remain complex and unrewarding, and their behavior may be viewed as either externalizing (defiant, eliciting rejection or punitive responses) or internalizing (depressed, sad, distant, withdrawn, or fatigued). Processing trauma is very necessary, and children have their own particular ways of achieving a resolution as well as learning more adaptive coping strategies. Dynamic posttraumatic play decreases the intensity of the trauma by giving children exposure opportunities (expressive release). The therapeutic outcomes indicate that they have received and accepted help and may be more capable of doing other kinds of work because their avoidance has been overcome. Marans, Mayes, and Colonna (1993), cited in Cohen et al. (2010), make an important statement: "Play activity functions in various ways to help the young child rework unpleasant experiences, gain self-efficacy, reduce arousal, make negative experiences more predictable and recreate meaning from overwhelming chaos" (p. 162).

When posttraumatic play is dynamic, treatment progresses and children improve in their ability to have relational success, their willingness to reach out to attachment figures, and their capacity for self-soothing and regulation; as a result, they achieve a renewed sense of confidence and competence. Posttraumatic play advances therapy goals and may prepare children for additional services such as group and family therapy, or specific techniques such as trauma-focused cognitive-behavioral therapy (TFCBT), eye movement desensitization and reprocessing (EMDR), or equine-assisted therapy. Such approaches may become more palatable to children who initially resist direct work or are too dysregulated for cognitive work. Bruce Perry has advocated for sequential therapies that target different parts of the brain, arguing that all therapeutic approaches have their merit, but the timing of their delivery and their focus on altering brain patterns should be of utmost priority (Perry & Dobson, 2013). I believe that children have ample opportunities to self-soothe, challenge their defenses, and explore the nature of trust within relationships by participating in child-centered play therapy first, allowing for the emergence of posttraumatic play which provides management of trauma through self-initiated exposure techniques.

When posttraumatic play is dynamic, it is less about clinical technique and more about providing the self of the therapist as an object of security and trust. The more clinicians can become trustworthy and emotionally present to anchor the therapy relationship, the better. I have great optimism about what the child can accomplish under these circumstances, while heeding the warning that posttraumatic play can become dangerous to the child and needs constant monitoring.

The intent of posttraumatic play is to restore personal power and control, which is usually compromised during traumatic experiences. Maria Fernanda's response to a catastrophic earthquake, described earlier, illustrates how dynamic posttraumatic play (especially in combination with a supportive, empathic parent) produces the child's renewed experience of mastery as its best possible outcome. When assessing the type and extent of traumatic impact in children, clinicians are best informed by the traumatized individuals themselves and the degree of debilitating helplessness they endured. The key factor seems to be whether the event overwhelmed the person's perceived ability to cope, causing the person to feel helpless, hopeless, distrustful, or filled with acute fear and sometimes emotional (and physical) paralysis. During experiences of extreme fear and arousal, the brain emits adrenalin and cortisol, chemicals that can cause physical changes in strength and mobility. The individual experiences immediate and acute changes in breathing, pulse rate, physical responses, and feeling state. Some people experiencing trauma have noted that they were either unable to move or propelled into action, running distances quickly or lifting heavy objects or pushing through barriers. It's unclear what variables influence whether individuals respond by fighting, fleeing, or freezing. Just as a defensive strategy may be physiologically driven and less consciously chosen, so the avenue by which traumatized individuals manage traumatic experiences is varied and unpredictable.

I have always wondered why some children can readily access and make use of posttraumatic play while other children cannot. This question seems comparable to why children in distress develop either internalized or externalized behaviors, although parental modeling, genetics, temperament and personality, prior stressors, and gender may influence the formation of their symptoms, defensive mechanisms, and coping strategies.

TOXIC POSTTRAUMATIC PLAY: THE NEGATIVE ASPECT

Terr (1991) became fascinated with posttraumatic play during her longitudinal study of children who were kidnapped in Chowchilla, California. In addition to carefully specifying the characteristics of this play described in Chapter 1, she cautioned about a retraumatizing kind of play:

> But play does not stop easily when it is traumatically inspired. And it may not change much over time. As opposed to ordinary child's play, post-traumatic play is obsessively repeated. It is grim. Furthermore, it requires a certain set of conditions in order to proceed: a certain place, a certain assortment of dolls, certain playmates, or a certain routine. It may go on for years. It repeats parts of the trauma. It occasionally includes a defense or two or a feeble attempt at a happy ending, but post-traumatic play is able to do very little to relieve anxiety. It can be dangerous, too. The problem is post-traumatic play may create more terror than was consciously there when the game started. And if it does dissipate some terror, this monotonous play does it so slowly that it might take more than a lifetime before the play would completely dissipate all the anxiety stirred up by the trauma. (p. 239)

MICKEY: AN EXAMPLE OF TOXIC POSTTRAUMATIC PLAY

Mickey was 7 when I first met him. He had been sexually abused by a transient, homeless person whom his mother befriended and provided childcare for him. Mickey and his mother had a history of homelessness and of moving around from state to state. The department of family services (DFS) had identified this family as high risk and had placed them in a hotel until they could help secure them more permanent housing. A social worker had recently begun to assess the mother's strengths and vulnerabilities and whether she was receptive to concrete services that would help her provide safe and consistent care for her child.

Mickey was very dysregulated with a host of symptomatic behaviors that signaled his distress and his acute fear and anxiety. He rarely slept through the night, he had night terrors and sonambulism, and he was aggressive to peers as well as to adults. In school he could not sit still, popping in and out of his chair wandering around the room, and he had left the school premises twice. He needed persistent and intense monitoring to get him safely through the day. Two schools had expelled him because they felt he was a danger to himself and others. In addition to behaviors directed at others, Mickey hit his head against the wall, set small fires, frequently holding his fingers to the flame, and took very hot showers. He focused a lot of negative behaviors on his mother, hitting her, biting her, and pushing her against the wall. Their size difference did not mediate his ability to impose himself on his mother, and she seemed passive and helpless in response to his aggression. Not surprisingly, we later discovered that his mother had a long and painful history of domestic violence and early physical and sexual abuse.

In therapy, Mickey was highly dysregulated for the first couple of months. He wanted to push me around, he spit on me, and he banged his head against the wall so hard that the hanging on the wall fell down, causing even him to startle—he was usually oblivious to the consequences of his behavior. His behavior required that limits be set almost every 10 minutes of each of our therapy sessions. Eventually, we negotiated a set of consequences that worked for us both. He got one warning, and if he could not regulate himself, he got one more. The third warning signaled the termination of the session, and he had to be taken home early. Luckily, there were sufficient motivators for him to stay in the room: He liked a dart game that I had in the office, and he enjoyed throwing nerf darts at it. He also liked to play catch, although we had to switch from a football to a round ball when he kept throwing the ball so hard I couldn't catch it and it hit me. Therapy was a tough go; none of my usual interventions worked, and trust was quite difficult to establish. I don't think Mickey ever learned to trust me, although he did eventually grow to rely on the fact that I would not hurt him physically, emotionally, or verbally (no matter how creative his behavior) and, unlike his mother, I would not let him hurt me. The first two or three months I literally held my breath when I went out to the waiting room to find him. His dysregulation would be low, moderate, or severe, but it was always present. What struck me the most was how he set up situations in which he was the aggressor or the victim. He always tried to "get my goat" by calling me names, spitting, taking apart and breaking toys, or smearing paints or chalks on my clothes. It was as if he was constantly checking to see if I would react to him the way almost everyone else did, with rudeness, with aggression, or with dismissive behavior.

I was patient. I got special consultation, and I received him warmly each time, expecting that each new session might be different and that he might feel better or less upset. Those hopes quickly faded as we reached the midpoint of our sessions. I decided to make his session a little longer to give him more time in that small window when he would take a breath and settle in. I also increased his time to twice a week for a while (which was counterintuitive to him) to give him a chance to become more comfortable with me. I paid the price for adding a second weekly session at first, but eventually he relented ever so slightly. These early sessions are now a blur. It mostly felt like an exercise in mindfulness and radical acceptance. Being with him was very challenging, and it took a great deal of energy for me to resist taking his bait. Eventually, he protested less and participated more. At about the fifth month, which coincided with summer, we returned to a weekly schedule, and he was quite pleased. By this time, he had asked for specific types of toys (super-heroes and villains), and I had ordered those for my miniature collection. This is one of the first times I remember sitting with an iPad, ordering precisely the toys a child client wanted (within very specific limits). I can no longer remember the names of these characters; suffice to say that the villains were quite well defined, the stories elaborate and fluid, and the heroes tireless. Mickey never touched the sand in the sandbox; however, he asked for the sand to be taken out of the tray and wanted an empty box in which to create and narrate his stories (later he called the empty sandbox his "work space").

Mickey's posttraumatic play emerged quickly. He set up a scenario in which one small figure was beaten, stabbed, and "raped" (his word) by at least 20 villains. He used soldiers to help the villains do more damage to the victim. The beatings were intense, and he went into a dissociative state and seemed to break a sweat. When he plummeted a soldier's sword into the buttocks of the victim, he touched himself frequently and seemed to get an erection. He always went to the bathroom during this play, and I suspected that walking to the bathroom gave him a chance to break out of his dissociative state. He always went to the bathroom at the same place in the sequence of his play, after shoving the weapon into the victim's buttocks a number of times. He would always come back with water on his face and red cheeks. He could not volunteer any information about this play, and when I described the sequence of the play to him (a simple behavioral description of what I saw), he looked away and would not engage with me. The play always lasted approximately 25 minutes, and during that time he was intensely focused and noninteractive. When I checked with his foster parent to see how he was doing, she commented that he was "impossible and out of control" when he got home from therapy and picked a fight with everyone. It concerned me that she said he was regressing back to the behaviors he had exhibited when he had first been placed. I was having a different experience with him as he was focused and attentive to his play in-session, but his dysregulation at home and school continued to be problematic.

This is a perfect example of posttraumatic play that is toxic and does not cause relief. This type of posttraumatic play can actually exacerbate symptoms and gives the impression that it is stuck through its repetition and rigidity. This negative posttraumatic play must be stopped through carefully structured directive interventions. In Chapter 4 I discuss appropriate interventions in toxic posttraumatic play, but as readers can assess from the case I have described, this play does not meet its intended goal of mastery and keeps children feeling retraumatized and "stuck" in problem interactions and behaviors. In cases of dynamic play, although behaviors or emotional problems may be exacerbated as the play becomes intensely repetitive, eventually, as the play enters a phase of reparation, symptoms decrease and the child becomes stable. In dynamic posttraumatic play, I take a more child-centered approach, I follow the child's lead. When toxic posttraumatic play occurs, I take charge and provide the necessary external guidance to help the play move along in a more productive fashion.

As noted, posttraumatic play can become unproductive and retraumatizing and may lead to negative outcomes, but I have seen some remarkable outcomes of this play with direct clinical interventions. Chapter 3 offers specific ideas for optimizing dynamic posttraumatic play and preventing or interrupting toxic patterns.

FORMS OF POSTTRAUMATIC PLAY

Terr emphasizes that children can express their trauma through post-traumatic play or through behavioral enactments. In this section, I discuss four variations of posttraumatic play and reenactment: (1) the use of objects to literally represent a specific trauma, (2) symbolic posttraumatic play that disguises the trauma specifics, (3) posttraumatic behavioral reenactments by the child playing alone, and (4) posttraumatic reenactments by the child attempting to enlist others in reenactments. Engaging others in reenactments of interpersonal complex trauma (Type II) is particularly tricky and can pose personal risks to young children whose behaviors can be misinterpreted and mislabeled. A brief example of each of these variations of posttraumatic play follows.

MICHAEL: AN EXAMPLE OF LITERAL POSTTRAUMATIC PLAY

Five-year-old Michael was severely neglected and occasionally physically abused. His play was a literal description of his numerous traumas at the hands of his parents. From the moment he entered his first session, he grabbed a small male figurine, a mother and father, and a baby brother. He looked at me with the toys in his hands and said, "This is Daddy; he's not here. This is Mommy; she's tired. And this is Bobby; he's mine." From that moment, he showed precisely what had occurred in his home. He would say, "The fridge is empty, just old milk," or "Bobby pooed in his diapers but no more diapers here," or "My mom is sleeping and she drank all the beer." All the various and disturbing aspects of his neglect and abuse were on vivid display as Michael moved his toy figures around and told stories about how "the big brother" had taken care of "the little brother," put him to sleep, and gone next door for milk when his brother wouldn't stop crying. (Amazingly, one of Michael's neighbors was aware the two boys were alone and would check in on them and bring food from time to time, but she never called the police, stating she wouldn't "turn in" her friend.) While playing with his toys, Michael would often have the father doll return to the house and "spank the mom" for falling asleep. Sometimes, in his compensatory stories, his father would take Michael and Bobby out to the park. Other times, Michael would go to school and have friends who would invite him to their houses for dinner. The stories were heartbreaking, and yet it was clear that Michael was externalizing and subsequently facing all the parenting deficits evident in his mother (and father), as well as his reactions and responses to his chaotic environment. As the play continued and evolved, it was evident that Michael was attempting to create resources and possibilities, and learning to express his fears, wishes, and worries. This child and his brother were eventually reunited with their father after 2 years in foster care. During that time, social service professionals did their best to educate the father, assist him in securing housing, employment, and childcare. Most importantly, Michael and Bobby's father seemed to mature and make good use of the services he was provided. Their mother, however, fell deeper into a spiral of drugs and despair, as a result of which her parental rights were terminated, a fact that affected Michael but not Bobby, who could barely remember her. When Michael and Bobby's father remarried, the professional team felt great optimism about the good choice the father had made and the investment that his new wife made in the children.

Michael selected and named his family members while first calling himself "the big brother." Eventually, he mustered the courage to move into first-person descriptions of what he had seen, heard, thought, and felt. During his repetitive play, he showed how he was hungry, how he changed his brother's diapers and rocked him at night so he could sleep. He also showed his mother's inability to parent, and her absence was palpable. Most of the incidents of abuse in Michael's police report were shown through his very literal posttraumatic play, and new incidents also appeared. Most importantly, Michael's resiliency, strength, courage, and tender caretaking also appeared. He often stated that he liked his "new mom and dad," and he hoped he could live with them "always." As a reunification process began with his father, Michael's play softened to a more empathic and consistent father.

AN EXAMPLE OF SYMBOLIC POSTTRAUMATIC PLAY

Ten-year-old Rocio was sexually abused by her mother's boyfriend. The abuse always happened when her mother left them alone to go to work. Rocio had begged her mother to please take her to work with her, but she repeatedly left Rocio alone with her boyfriend. She later said she was unaware of the danger. Rocio told her teacher that she didn't like being at home alone when her mother went to work and eventually confided why. This disclosure was handled seriously with an immediate call to child protective services (CPS), which placed the child in an emergency foster home. CPS referred the call to the police, who interviewed Rocio and asked her to participate in a phone sting which Rocio did, though with trepidation. When she called the house to tell her mother's boyfriend that she was staying with a friend after school, he became irate and told her it was important for them to have their special time. The child was coached to talk to him so that he admitted what he was doing to her; upon this admission, he was immediately arrested.

Rocio was incredibly avoidant and frightened. She was a native Spanish-speaker, but somehow my speaking Spanish made her more uncomfortable. She was afraid of her mother, it turned out, and was terrified that she would pay for talking to others about the "secret game," which she had already shared with her mother. This was one of those rare cases in which the mother knew what was going on but felt it was more important for her to go to work than to try to protect her child. The mother later told me that she had been abused all her childhood years and that she had just "learned to ignore it." This might have been the mother's primitive description of having learned to dissociate and expecting her daughter to do the same.

Rocio selected the following toys: a large, white bear that she named "Mami Lily." It was interesting that she chose a white mother bear who lay playfully on her back. For herself, she chose a small brown bear, who had a colorful block in its hands, and a large black bird which was landing with his claws ready to grab prey. She also included a large angel figure that held a magnifying glass. Rocio confided that this angel was a grandmother who would never let anything bad happen to the baby bear.

The entire narrative was orchestrated with the symbols Rocio chose. She never placed these items in a dollhouse, and she always played sitting on the floor. She also never called these toys her mother, herself, her grandmother, or her mother's boyfriend, but these identities were understood and implied in the way she spoke about them. The mother was always out of sight, busy playing and on her back. The bird was always hovering, ready to attack as soon as the mother bear left. The angel said her prayers, and the little bear "wants to be alone and play baby games." Rocio eventually testified in court, and the offender was convicted. The mother's parental rights were terminated, and Rocio was adopted by a large family with two sisters and two brothers. At a later juncture, she participated in group therapy for youngsters with histories of abuse, and she participated openly and without reservation. It was clear to her by then that her mother was neglectful, that the offender was sick, and that she was not to blame for what had happened. All those realizations occurred through her symbolic play and without my making definitive interpretations. She designated the large hovering bird as "cruel" and "too hungry." The baby bear would get carried away and hidden by the angel. Other times, Mami Lily would take a shotgun and, laughing, would shoot at the bird. This bird circled over and over without words, but Rocio made the squawking sounds of the bird, the gunshot sounds, and the whimpering and giggling of the mother bear who was on her back. At one point, the baby bear tried to help the mother stand up, but the mother refused, saying that she had other things to do. Thus, Rocio's play was relentlessly repetitive. Without using names or taking ownership of the characters, she managed to work through her experiences of helplessness, vulnerability, fear, and loneliness. Of course, living in a safe setting contributed greatly to her sense of security and growing confidence. As the play progressed, Rocio also found a small duck friend for her bear, and they eventually took outings. She also buried the scary bird under sand and stated she would "never see him more!" These changes were reflective of the new experiences she was actively welcoming into her life.

GABE: AN EXAMPLE OF INDIVIDUAL POSTTRAUMATIC BEHAVIORAL REENACTMENTS

Five-year-old Gabe was held down in a bathtub until he could not breathe. This "lesson" from his father had been repeated several times. The father had been taught right and wrong by his own father using this horrific parenting "technique." On one of those occasions,

Gabe struggled against his father, hit his head on the water faucet, and had to be taken to the hospital for stitches. The doctors made a definitive and swift report, and the child was given an emergency placement until the situation could be evaluated. The child's therapy with me proceeded well, and it was a matter of weeks before he asked if he could show me that he had made "water bullets" by immersing paper towels in water. He told me that his foster mother had asked him to stop doing this play at home but asked him to show me in therapy. His foster mother had called me beforehand to mention the child's interest in this specific play, so in preparation I brought a roll of paper towels and water into the office. Gabe was thrilled to see that he would be allowed to play freely; he pulled out the paper towel pieces, scrunched them into big bunches, and pushed them into a small pitcher containing water. After doing this, he pulled them out, molded them into smaller balls, and asked to throw them against the wall. He was very excited when I suggested we take this game outside where he could use a large brick wall as a target for his water balls. "Splat, splat," the wet towel balls would sound as he threw them against the wall. He seemed to get more and more actively involved with the process of throwing the towels each time. He began to look like a baseball pitcher, taking a big wind-up and sending the wet towel balls into the wall. When he was done, he looked relaxed and happy. This play took a few more turns. He went from paper towels to sponges and immersed sponges into a water bucket. Each time he would hold the sponges down carefully for a specific period of time. I timed this activity and found that each immersion lasted 35 seconds. He would always take a deep breath when he took the paper towels, and later the sponges, out of the water. Later, he immersed crystals and asked permission to throw them against the wall outside. I hesitated but compromised with a specific number of crystals. He chose only one color, baby blue. He took 10 of them and blasted them into the wall, shattering most of them. The end of this session included our picking up as many of the pieces as we could find and putting them into the trash. After this play, he moved on to different play activities and eventually engaged in both symbolic and conversational activities about his ambivalent feelings about his father, as well as the mother who waited outside the bathroom while father implemented his water-boarding.

This child and his father participated in some effective reconciliatory family therapy that included a period of therapy for dad, which led to his realization that his water technique constituted child abuse. He delivered a sincere apology for scaring and hurting his son. With the monitoring of CPS, ongoing home-based therapy, and our family therapy sessions, father and mother were exposed to new, healthier, and safer disciplinary techniques, and the child thrived. The parents opted to divorce a year later, and Gabe chose to live with his mother (with father's consent), with regular visitation with dad.

Gabe's play had a physical and sensory component that allowed him to release some of the fear and anger he had stored. His holding his breath during the immersions of his towels and the vast breath he released were reminiscent of the abuse he had endured. As he played, he took an active role that permitted abreaction and physical release.

The question of whether to offer a clinical interpretation that connects the play to the actual events continues to be a subject of lively discussion. However, I trust that children understand on a deep level the play that they create. I believe that as they invest themselves in playing, they are actively engaged in activating their whole person. On occasion, when I have attempted to draw comparisons, children quickly deny the correlation; they seem to feel inhibited and then are suddenly uninterested in their play. For this reason, and because of my trust in the process, I prefer to let children arrive at their own understanding as they interact with their play. That's not to say that I don't also interact with the play, ask amplifying questions, or reflect to children what I see them do. In other words, there are ample clinical responses that I might employ. Interpretation can be a disruptive factor for children, although I'm sure the therapist's comfort and trust in this technique make a huge difference in how it is delivered and received.

MAGGIE: AN EXAMPLE OF ENGAGING OTHERS
IN POSTTRAUMATIC BEHAVIORAL REENACTMENTS

One of my earliest cases was with Maggie, a young girl of 8, who had been severely physically abused and had developed many of the characteristics of abused children: She was hypervigilant, fearful, compliant, avoidant, and always tried to please. After 5 or 6 months of therapy, this child brought a ping-pong paddle to the session and offered it to me. After asking her what it was and her responding the obvious, I asked her why she was giving it to me. She responded that it was for me to hit her. When I asked what made her think that I would hit her, she said, "You like me, don't you?" I was stunned by her explanation, and it took me a while to fully appreciate how her bringing me the paddle and asking to be hit was a sign of her negotiating her anxiety. This child was so unaccustomed to positive interactions with others that her anxiety had grown even as she concurrently experienced small levels of trust in me. Once her trust grew and she suspected that I cared for her, her next immediate concern was staying safe from what she expected would be a sudden change in my behavior. She had grown to believe that caring and violence were interwoven, and thus if I liked her (and she felt cared for), she would get hurt. Rather than tolerate the anxiety of this internal world view, she brought me the weapon so that I could act violently and then move on to the familiar postviolence phase of reconciliation. This was my first exposure to posttraumatic behavioral reenactment and to how powerful a force it can be. Needless to say, clinical responses must be clear and swift, so that children believe and trust that hurting will not be optional in the therapy relationship.

These types of posttraumatic play and behavior are all powered differently, and yet they seem designed to externalize the difficult or painful memories (sometimes experienced as feelings, sensations, vague thoughts, or mental pictures). Through utilizing posttraumatic play, children have the opportunity to decrease the intensity of their trauma responses and to assign more correct meanings to them. This working through of traumas through posttraumatic play allows children to face powerful memories through play, symbolic or literal, or through actual experience alone or with others.

There is no single explanation of how posttraumatic play or behavior is useful for children. My professional experience has taught me to suspend assumptions and simply await the next creative variation that each child can bring. I remain in awe of the self-reparative qualities of traumatized children when given the optimal environment, safety, respect, and support that includes parents and/

or caretakers, helping professionals, teachers, daycare providers, social workers, and the like.

PHASES OF POSTTRAUMATIC PLAY

Marvasti (1994) identified several stages of posttraumatic play, including diagnosis, relationship, and repetitive play. In each stage, he proposed a unique focus designed to assist the child's resulting empowerment. I have also observed stages or phases in children's posttraumatic play that appear to evolve over time in children who have experienced primarily Type II traumas. The following organizational schema may help clinicians observe specific and detectable phases and progression:

Externalization and Containment

In this earliest phase of posttraumatic play, the child commits to externalizing his or her worries and begins to select a literal or symbolic way of revealing known or still unknown thoughts, feelings, and reactions to the trauma experience. The child conducts an exploration in front of an unconditionally accepting witness, who is sometimes challenged and tested by children before, during, or after they externalize their play. During this phase of posttraumatic play, the child narrows his or her focus that gives way to clinical understanding. Throughout, the child exerts control—a necessary requisite for feeling safe. Clinicians utilizing a child-centered approach will find their witness role facile and comforting, trusting the child's process. However, children may leave the therapy office feeling tentative, tense, activated, energized, or emotionally constricted.

Release of Energy and Activation of Resources

In the middle phase of posttraumatic play, clinicians can observe sudden, sporadic, or growingly consistent movement and energy. What might have been rote and repetitive posttraumatic play in the first phase now morphs into play that includes small or large movements in storyline, characters, situations, beginnings or endings, and so on. The child in play may also look more physically fluid, vibrant, energetic, or engaged in a sensory way, making noises, physical movements, and taking up more room. The child is infusing the play with projection, as well as "news" about options, opportunities, and difference. The child moves from a position of passivity or tension to one of control and release. At this time, expression can become more ample, although the smallest sign of release (e.g., a sigh) must be recognized. The child also seems to self-regulate and self-soothe, and becomes capable of stopping the play and keeping the end-time of the session in mind. Children usually do not leave the play unhappy or tense, but may develop symptoms at home or school.

Age-Appropriate Resolution and Closure

During this final phase of posttraumatic play, the child appears to have a greater sense of confidence and may be experiencing mastery in his or her play. During this phase, the child may have asserted certain beliefs and may gain a deeper understanding of why things happened. Children appear to have a period of introspection, which sometimes is followed by their giving voice to their characters, asking questions, making statements, or being more responsive to clinical queries to amplify the metaphors they have presented. The final goal of crafting a narrative that is organized and more clearly defined (either in symbolic or literal fashion) is achieved. The child appears relieved and more receptive to other interventions, such as cognitive reassessment and processing. Children may leave therapy with mixed emotions, initially unsettled. However, with some forms of resolution come tranquility and closure.

One additional factor bears mention and can often cause clinical concern. As mentioned earlier, not all children utilize posttraumatic play, and not every child follows a structured course of posttraumatic play. For some children it is consistently repetitive and driven; for others it is more sporadic, appearing at intervals. In these cases, children may be pacing themselves, gathering forces so to speak. Even more importantly, some children appear to have dissociative responses to their play. I have consulted with many clinicians who become alarmed when this occurs. Dissociation is highly linked to trauma and serves as an important defensive strategy in which children compartmentalize and suspend the immediacy of their painful external stressor. Children are fiercely creative, often "going out of body," numbing out parts of their body, or depersonalizing. It makes sense to me that the gradual exposure inherent in posttraumatic play will trigger familiar defensive responses in children. In my experience, dissociative states are common when children are engaged in dynamic or toxic posttraumatic play and sometimes when they are engaged in solitary or peer reenactments of trauma.

Even when children are dissociating during these activities, and go in and out of altered states of consciousness, they are causing some change to occur. Dissociation could emerge during play or reenactment as a reminder of dissociative states during the actual abuse, or as a defensive response to the play or behavior they initiate. I regard this as part of the recovery process and not a definitive negative, as long as children are able to come in and out of dissociative states, and the episodes become shorter in length over time. There are times when I might attempt to interrupt pervasive dissociation by taking a more active role (Gil, 1989), and this requires a departure from the actual play.

HOW POSTTRAUMATIC PLAY HELPS HEAL

By definition, play provides a protective cushion for children. It allows them to distance themselves from traumatic memories while externalizing them, so that they can be viewed as much or as little as can be tolerated. As children expose themselves to concrete images reminiscent of traumatic memories, their feelings are evoked and hopefully, the beginning of management occurs. Maria Fernanda, for example, did a number of different things: She dug small holes in the dirt, and she buried dead bugs in the dirt. We might therefore consider whether she was facing the fact that the earth had swallowed up her uncle. Once buried, would she help him out? She did not, but she did place live bugs in the dirt, who could make their way out. Likely, she had hoped that her uncle would miraculously find his way out of the earth or would be discovered some day. These were not conscious processes for Maria Fernanda, and she was unable to answer her mother's simple questions about the play or accept her ideas about why she was playing with the dirt. This kind of play is not always rational, but it makes sense in the context of what the child has experienced and may be trying to resolve. It is important to note that Maria Fernanda initiated posttraumatic play on the same day of the week that the earthquake that killed her uncle occurred. These anniversary behaviors are not often consciously chosen.

CONCLUSION

Posttraumatic play is a creative mechanism designed by children to accomplish gradual exposure (Gil, 2013). As such, it allows traumatized children to gradually see, feel, express, release, and mediate traumatic memories. By playing, they slowly but surely organize their memories, and they begin to have a reparative experience that inevitably results in an improved and restored sense of mastery and personal control. Posttraumatic play provides a distancing mechanism that allows children to "own" their difficult memories gradually and to attempt to manage their underlying, often unspoken, concerns. Thus, they may use symbols or metaphors to communicate about themselves and others, negating ownership of thoughts and feelings that cannot be expressed, and at the same time acknowledging and tolerating them. When children begin to feel stronger and less helpless, they may suddenly need less distance and can shift from symbolic play to more realistic play in which they assert ownership and articulate the thoughts and feelings they could only hint about earlier. Often this play is a type of rehearsal, a testing of the water that can precede meaningful change.

Clinical attention to posttraumatic play has unconditional acceptance and witnessing as a basic foundation, which allows clinicians to provide necessary directive and nondirective responses while observing the natural evolution of the play.

Ideally, posttraumatic play results in a renewed sense of power and control, the development of an organized narrative, and the release or expression of physical or emotional responses associated with the traumatic events. It can help children to grow in confidence and to reestablish their sense of trust in others through a course of treatment that is trauma-focused and relational and that values, allows, or encourages the child's posttraumatic play.

By miniaturizing events that loom large in the child's mind or body, the child begins to face the intolerable by moving the toy objects, giving them a voice, and becoming the change agent of the traumatic memory. The child moves from a passive stance of victim to the more active stance of someone who is in charge. Children can take in the miniaturized or symbolized scene, and they hold the power to make necessary changes in the storyline. These are two of the restorative elements of posttraumatic play. Infusing toy objects with the ability to move, take action, make noises, object, make demands, or scold greatly contributes to self-reparation. It's also likely that playing in front of an accepting witness who is engaged and empathic as ugly trauma secrets are revealed also seems to create a helpful, relational context. As hurtful truths are revealed, and checked out with witnesses through a glance or grunt, resources may be accessed and incorporated into the play. In the final transformative phase of post-traumatic play, the child may introduce heroes and protective parents or other adults, and may even weave in some aspect of the therapy or therapist.

Posttraumatic play that is toxic requires a more active and directive clinical approach. It will be important for therapists to be patient, well informed, and prepared to intervene when necessary. Yes, posttraumatic play can become repetitive, ritualistic, disguised, or joyless, but it needs time to be unpackaged, aired, and infused with new energy, perspective, or expression of affect. In this way, it can afford the player a tremendous opportunity for reparation.

The next chapter provides therapists with relevant information about how to observe and document posttraumatic play, evaluate which type of posttraumatic play the child is using, and determine what clinical responses to provide. Ideas for intervening in toxic post-traumatic play are also presented.

3

Evaluating Posttraumatic Play and Intervening When It Is Toxic

*I*n my experience, many children spontaneously use posttraumatic play, whereas other children need encouragement and reinforcement. Herein lies the clinical dilemma: How do clinicians know if the play is helpful or not? What are the differentiating characteristics of dynamic and toxic posttraumatic play, and what clinical interventions are needed if the play is not serving its projected purpose?

MATT: AN EXAMPLE OF DYNAMIC POSTTRAUMATIC PLAY

Matt was a 9-year-old with a history of neglect and sexual abuse. He had been abused by an unrelated male, formerly his mother's boyfriend. He had been removed from the home when his mother persisted in putting her children in harm's way. She would often send them outside the apartment building when she was scoring drugs. The children were viewed as unsupervised by police and placed in different foster homes. The mother went in and out of drug rehab programs, and Matt was fortunate to find a permanent foster home where he lived until he was 21.

Matt's presentation was the polar opposite of Mickey's (described in Chapter 2). Matt was compliant and passive, with lowered eyes and a soft voice. He constantly squirmed in his chair and was constricted in his movements and emotional expressions. I mirrored his quiet demeanor at first, focused on getting him to know me and the environment. His foster parent had told me that he was "never a bother," and often she "didn't know he was there." I recognized his attempts to be invisible as an adaptive behavior in children who experience or witness violence. He wanted to stay out of sight so that he could feel safe. He had learned to make himself small and to keep out of the way. He was definitely not able to be himself, and I spent the first two months doing parallel play, making few demands of him to participate in specific activities, and developing predictable beginnings and endings. By the fourth month of therapy, Matt looked up more frequently, volunteered information, and was able to laugh and ask for specific activities. There was very little limit-setting with this child, and his overpoliteness and helpfulness were signs of fear, mistrust, and lack of security. In the fourth month, he turned his attention to the sandbox that he had ignored in all prior sessions. He began a very slow and purposeful type of play that eventually I recognized as posttraumatic play. This case has been documented elsewhere (Gil, 2006b), but suffice it to say here that he brought his sexual abuse into the therapy office by using a miniaturized story that clearly showed what had happened to him and gave him a chance to regain control. His play was measured and resolute: He spent at least six to eight sessions with his hands in the box, patting, pushing, stirring, drawing with a finger, and finally, in each session, restoring the sand to its original shape. Midway, he found water appealing, and he wet the tray a little, enough to be able to continue his patting, pushing, and stirring. Eventually, his play transitioned into his making small mounds with his hands, cupping them into a perfect shape, each mound exactly like the other. Once he perfected six perfectly consistent mounds, he used his fingers to make an opening at the top, resembling volcanoes. He would frequently flatten them after making eye contact with me, to check whether I had seen what he did. I remember saying things like "You are patting the sand just like you want to," or "You've got just the right amount of water in there," or "You've made these mounds look perfectly alike." He always acknowledged my talking to him, but he never responded verbally. It was as if he was gathering his strength for what was to come, an insight I had well after the fact.

Eventually, the mounds with the openings elicited active play from Matt, and he opened his body, bringing his arms around in large circles with small airplanes in his hands. He would make the planes fly around, until finally they would crash into the holes, burying half the plane in the mound. The planes would remain in these mounds, as if stuck. There was always some small visible reaction in Matt when he finished this play and listened to my descriptive statements. Then he would take the airplanes out, throw them on the floor (which was unlike him), and gently push together the opening, restoring the mound to its former shapes. He would then begin to slowly move the sand around, destroying the mounds, and flattening the sand before leaving. This restoration of the sand to its previously flat, untouched, serene state might have been evidence of his trust that reparation to a pre-abuse state of calm (and innocence) was possible. I described this sequential behavior back to him: He always nodded in agreement.

Matt had been sodomized precisely six times, and it became evident to me that he was reenacting the intrusive assaults over and over. But the healing seemed to occur in the removing of the planes and discarding them, as well as the tender caretaking he seemed to give the mounds as he repaired the openings and replaced the sand to its flat state, patting it down as if to say, "There, there." I noticed that Matt's demeanor changed during this time. His compliance seemed to change some, and he would take more initiative with his foster parents. He volunteered more information to me and others, and his caved-in chest began to open. He explored the room after his sand play, and he smiled from time to time. One day he laughed fully at something silly that I said. His laughter was music to my ears. About four months later, we viewed a psychoeducational video about a boy who had been abused by an older male. Matt sat next to me and held the remote control. I had told him to stop the tape whenever he wanted, and he did. When he stopped it, he would whisper to me about his mother's boyfriend, Freaky Frank, who had hurt him "lots of times." He said that after the man hurt him, Matt went into the bathroom and sat alone, washing himself with wet toilet paper, hoping he would not come into the bathroom to find him. He also told me that he closed his eyes and pretended that his mother came and found him in the bathroom, took him to the doctor, and then told the man to go away. Once he said to me, "But she never did, and she kept leaving me with him." He had made a mark in the bathroom for every time the abuse occurred. Later on in therapy, his play included lots of medical equipment in which he (the doctor) would examine kids "all over" and put Band-Aids over most of the dolls' bodies. "How did this happen to you?" and "Is someone hurting you?" were frequent questions, to which the dolls would respond "No."

It is sometimes mystifying to watch children achieve a sense of mastery through their play. When this happens, the noticeable outcome is that the children begin to express their thoughts and feelings (verbally or though expressive arts), feel more relaxed and confident, and appear better able to organize and show a narrative about their experience. In the play, they control what they see and what the clinician sees. They engage in repetition that allows them to discharge affect and gradually view and understand what they experienced. Sometimes they share verbally and sometimes they don't, but their play changes, as does their behavior in and out of session. Dynamic posttraumatic play has ample positive effects when it accomplishes its intended goal.

DISTINGUISHING TOXIC FROM DYNAMIC POSTTRAUMATIC PLAY

Matt's and Mickey's case histories show how disparate posttraumatic play can be and suggest that differential clinical responses do become necessary. The basic differentiation between dynamic and toxic posttraumatic play relates to its usefulness to the child. Cohen et al. (2010) note that "strategies of reenactment with soothing represent adaptive play as described in Zero to Three (2005), whereas the strategies of overwhelming re-experiencing are significantly and negatively related to them, and represent maladaptive post-traumatic play" (p. 176). Posttraumatic play, she states, is "both an adaptive attempt on the part of the child, using one's own capacities to deal with traumatic events, and also as a sign of maladaptation, signaling the need for help" (p. 174).

In a study of 29 Israeli children who had been exposed to terrorism, Cohen et al. (2010) found that many of her subjects used "their own powers of imagination, narrative creation, and soothing" as a way to exhibit "natural resilience and the curative function of spontaneous play" (p. 177). My impression is that self-soothing and adaptation might translate into an experience of mastery for traumatized children.

Toxic posttraumatic play is retraumatizing and potentially dangerous for children because it keeps them feeling trapped and in pain. In this state, they view everything through the lens of trauma: relationships, friendships, requests, attempts to help, and they reject helpful interactions and activities designed to move them toward healing. This type of play also looks deceptively like dynamic posttraumatic play. The dilemma for clinicians is determining how long to maintain a child-centered approach and when and how to intervene in a more directive way. Dripchak (2007) states that "the risk of the negative type of post-traumatic play is that it may actually worsen the traumatic effects and cause developmental regression. The child needs help to move on" (p. 126).

Documenting Posttraumatic Play

Over the years, I learned that paying focused attention to the play, documenting the smallest details and chronicling sequential sessions of the play, constitute the best clinical approach. It is important to state here that not all posttraumatic play happens in consecutive sessions. As mentioned earlier, posttraumatic play may be evident in consecutive fashion, or there may be brief spurts of play followed by interruptions. Thus, the chronicling becomes necessary so that we don't overrely on what we remember. Simply put, the primary issues for documentation consist of watching for changes and movement in posttraumatic play. Dynamic posttraumatic play may start in a rigid and structured way, but it ultimately gives way to health-promoting features such as abreaction, ownership of the play, and possibly insight or spontaneous communication. Toxic play starts and remains rigid, with no introduction of change or movement of any type and no advancement in therapy. Children's symptoms often escalate during dynamic posttraumatic play and then subside, peaking and stabilizing. In toxic posttraumatic play, symptoms may remain consistent and/or may peak and remain exacerbated. There have been times when I have gently guided children away from posttraumatic play or behavioral reenactments, and introduced other activities such as relaxation techniques, biblio- and videotherapy, or peer therapy.

Guidelines for Assessing Types of Posttraumatic Play

The following guidelines may be helpful in assessing the type of play that is being employed by the child and selecting the best clinical interventions for each unique child and family

1. Consider using the Trauma Play Scale (Myers, Bratton, & Hagen, 2011) to establish a baseline of observable behaviors.

2. Use the Checklist for Posttraumatic Play (see the Appendix to help you identify most, if not all, aspects of the play and evaluate changes over time).

3. After each session, make a record of small or large changes in the play. Changes to assess are:

a. *How the child starts the play.* Is he or she focused and eager? Does he or she back into the play? Is the child excited to pick up where he or she left off? Is the child immediately disengaged and avoidant of interactions with the clinician? Does the child seem hesitant and hypervigilant prior to starting the play? Does the child set up a recognizable routine that precedes (and predicts) the play? Does he or she try to "sneak in" the play without being observed?

b. *Characters used, new inclusions or absence of others.* Children usually externalize the play using miniatures, puppets, or other symbolic material. Thus, it will be important to note whether chosen materials change in any way, whether some are hidden away, kept separate, sometimes included and other times kept out. The introduction and ejection of story characters are useful to note.

c. *Affective or personality changes in the characters.* Children utilize projection freely, infusing their symbols with emotions and verbalizations. Clinical observation of personality traits or affective states will be relevant, just as changes that occur over time.

d. *Verbal and nonverbal communication.* Some children are silent throughout posttraumatic play, and some are not. Often children don't use words but can use a range of sounds, grunts, and noises.

e. *Sequence of the play and whether variations occur.* Clinicians should take note of the sequence of play, that is, what happens first, second and third. The rigid repetition of the sequence will signal important variables in the play that could help determine whether or not intervention is necessary.

f. *Endings of the play and any different outcomes.* The ending of the "story" is quite germane to determining the health of the child. Sometimes endings can suggest that children are addressing or attempting to resolve challenging thoughts or feelings related to the trauma. In the endings, clinicians can identify areas of difficulty as well as areas of hope.

g. *Adding or deleting parts of the story.* Changes in the story can occur for different reasons and can be a sign of resilience or a sign of regression. Knowing that specific data are being withheld or included can promote clinical understanding of how the child is managing his or her traumatic stress.

h. *Interactions with the therapist.* I have had children direct me to "turn around" and not watch them while they are working. Other children have wanted me to watch intensely, so much so that they asked me to come closer and closer to the place where they were doing their primary work. Some children talk, others are silent. There is no "one way" for children to interact with the therapist, but I like to document baseline behavior during the whole session and subsequent changes during the play or at other times.

i. *Location of the play.* One of the major variables in posttraumatic play is *movement*. Keep in mind that any kind of movement (behavioral, affective, physical) can indicate progress toward health. For example, taking the play out of the sand tray and placing it in a dollhouse can be a huge shift.

j. *Play before and after the posttraumatic work.* What children do before and after the posttraumatic play is also worth documenting. How children prepare to do this work and how they take care of themselves afterward allow us to make clinical judgments about children's current functioning and needs.

k. *Dissociation.* Dissociative episodes should be noted with special care—in particular, where the episodes occur, how long they last, at what juncture, and how the child breaks the dissociative episode should be recorded. Depending on whether or not dissociative episodes become less frequent or less intense or shorter in duration, it might be relevant to bring these episodes to the child's attention. I have both had a discussion with children, labeling the behavior and citing how it can signal special issues or concerns, and I have video-taped sessions and shown the tapes to children, asking them to reflect on how they appear during dissociative states. Because dissociation is a learned defense that is developed over time and can later become activated by generalized stimulants, it is important to bring the control of dissociative responses back to the client. Children have told me how much they appreciate "spacing out when they want" versus "when it just takes over." Dissociative responses in children are important and expected trauma-related features that warrant clinical attention (Silberg, 2012).

4. Check in with caretakers between sessions to see how children are responding to attending therapy and engaging in posttraumatic play. In my experience, caretakers may report that children's problem behaviors or symptoms increase for a period of time before they stabilize and improve. I have always found that the escalation of behavioral or symptomatic concerns without relief after the posttraumatic play has emerged in therapy and is well underway can be a sign that the posttraumatic work is becoming toxic or unhelpful.

The National Child Traumatic Stress Network (NCTSN) cites several critical aspects of trauma-informed treatment, including the creation of safety and relational health, direct processing of traumatic material with cognitive reassessments and integration, exposure and integration of traumatic material, and future orientation (*www.nctsn.org*). It appears that posttraumatic play contributes to these overall goals in very positive ways.

INTERVENING IN TOXIC POSTTRAUMATIC PLAY

In cases of toxic posttraumatic play, direct and well-designed clinical interventions are necessary to assist traumatized children. If left unattended, toxic posttraumatic play is potentially retraumatizing and halts all therapeutic progress.

Once this negative type of play is identified, there is no single answer to the question "How long do I wait to intervene?" My suggestion, described earlier, is to assess whether or not children's posttraumatic play appears to be moving in the right direction, check in with caretakers to hear about children's behaviors and emotional state out of session, and of course carefully assess the child's overall progress in therapy, evaluating general or global functioning.

Over the years, through trial and error, I have developed an understanding of the underlying dynamics in toxic posttraumatic play. Though not conclusive or applicable to every child, these dynamics might shed some light on why posttraumatic play can pose obstacles and cause havoc.

The Underlying Dynamics of Toxic Posttraumatic Play

Posttraumatic play is first and foremost an externalization that allows children to establish a *safe enough distance* from actual traumatic experiences. Children may have uncomfortable feelings when they remember or think about the trauma or abuse. They may feel flooded by feelings of fear, shame, worry, sadness, confusion, or anger, to name a few. They usually feel helplessness. When those feelings are left unattended, they remain intense and problematic to young children. When traumatic memories are unprocessed, thinking about or remembering traumatic memories produces feelings so intense and painful that avoidance definitely makes sense. Thus, as one child said to me, "I don't want to talk about it, and I don't want to think about it. When I think about it, I feel horrible, and I'm not doing it!!"

Children affected by earlier traumas look for ways to self-protect, for something to help them feel safe and less exposed and vulnerable. I believe that posttraumatic play points children to an avenue through which they can find self-reparation in a less painful, more creative way. Children externalize their memories, associated feelings, perceptions, cognitions, and body sensations through play by projecting their feelings safely onto the toys or miniatures they select. For example, a child who is being beaten by his parent may look up to a super-hero figure and infuse it with the ability to fly into his parent's room, changing the parent from mean to nice! The child might have the super-hero talk to the child, revealing the child's hidden feelings of sadness or hurt. Children can utilize the "as-if" quality of play for personal disguise so that things can be revealed and processed. Children enter this type of play fully, often losing themselves in their metaphors and stories. I believe strongly that the insights that children can glean on their own are often more comforting (and create more self-esteem) than external interpretations. One child gave me a bright smile when she declared, "Wow, I can't believe that I figured that out! Feel free to share with other kids if you like." I love to see this kind of confidence grow before my eyes when children "get" something on their own. Projection is a wonderful mechanism for children to use, and they use it routinely through play.

Sometimes the safe distancing available through play is insufficient. The desired cushion of safety is not available to the child, and he or she begins to feel continuously upset and hurt. Sometimes the child abandons the play completely, but other times clinicians will notice compulsive repetition of play in an overly structured and rigid way. Children may have dissociative episodes during this play, while symptoms increase and self-regulation decreases. In addition, regressed behaviors may appear or reappear. These changes may indicate that instead of children remembering the traumatic experiences at a distance, through their play, they are experiencing revivification—that is, a reliving of the trauma, complete with sensations, sights, sounds, thoughts, perceptions, and feelings that occurred during the traumatic incident. Lieberman and van Horn (2004a) suggest the import of encouraging a differentiation between reliving and remembering:

> Children reenact the traumatic experience through action or through play and may become increasingly confused about remembering and re-experiencing the trauma. The treatment aims at increasing their capacity to make the connection between what they are feeling in the moment and the traumatic experience in the past, emphasizing the concrete differences between their subjective experience and their present surroundings. (p. 125)

When these full memories occur and yield ongoing traumatic impact, children activate familiar defensive mechanisms; the same physiological responses occur, causing further learned helplessness. Instead of children feeling a renewed sense of control by playing things out, retraumatization ensues. Obviously, this development is undesirable, counterproductive, and potentially dangerous, and interferes with healing.

Posttraumatic play has a sensory component: kids are touching, holding, and moving around the toys and miniatures. Their hands are busy, and their bodies and minds are by extension engaged in play. For some children, the sensory component may be what causes the play to feel too close, interfering with the necessary safe distance. The play is too close, too intimate, and too compelling, so children cannot step back far enough to be the observer–participant. Instead, they experience the event they are recalling in vivo. This destabilizes them and elicits an abundance of difficult emotions. Thus, dissociative experiences come into play as an effective way to self-protect. When the required safe-enough distance does not occur, the play can become stilted, overwhelming, and unhelpful. When this occurs, clinical interventions are needed.

A Continuum of Interventions

Toxic posttraumatic play has many distinguishing characteristics, the most noteworthy being the repetitive and systematized nature of the play. It sometimes hardly seems like play at all. Its driven quality is quite apparent and noticeable. Therefore, when clinical interventions are required, clinicians must cause some change to occur to *disrupt* the rigid trajectory of the play. When I've made the decision to intervene, I try to do so from least to most disruptive. But the reality is that clinical intervention is urgent for several reasons: children are hurting, and they are at risk of feeling pain—symptoms are the same or increasing, normal development is delayed, and caretakers and loved ones are frustrated and uncertain about what they can do to help. The positive and optimistic intent of posttraumatic play has been thwarted, and a positive outcome is no longer likely.

The first four interventions that I list in the following paragraphs have sometimes been successful. If child-centered play therapy has taken place up to this point, nondirective play therapists can use these first four interventions to set the stage for a shift in clinical activity, something beyond patient observation and unconditional acceptance.

Verbalizing Descriptive Statements

Clinicians can begin to narrate what they see children doing. At this stage, pure descriptive statements work best: "I see the nurse and doctor are examining the baby and the baby is crying." No interpretations are made, such as "The baby doesn't like what the doctor is doing," or "The baby is afraid of seeing the doctor." Sometimes simple narrations can cause a shift in children's play, but more often than not, it doesn't do the trick. I have had the experience of children stopping their play altogether and waiting until I'm done talking to restart their play from the very beginning.

Asking Children to Give Characters a Voice

If children have been telling a repetitive story either through action or verbal narration, clinicians can ask children to give voice to the characters in their play, thereby giving them opportunities to show how characters they have incorporated into their stories might think or feel.

Changing the Sequence of Play

Ask children to start the play midpoint or to set the play up at a particular point, asking them to "take it from here." Children engaged in toxic posttraumatic play don't usually like this intervention either, preferring to return to their original starting point and following suit with their play.

Requesting Physical Movement and Breathing

Clinicians can attempt to break into the rigidity of the physical, emotional, or situation in the play (including dissociation at times) by having children move their bodies, breathe, and mobilize. Having children make the figure eight with their arms, reach both arms toward the sky one at a time, or take deep, cleansing breaths, can be helpful, sometimes leading the children to return to the play in an altered state that might produce a difference in perspective or behavior as well as in their interaction with the clinician.

I have found that more directive techniques are useful in interrupting posttraumatic play. Here are three of the most useful interventions; perhaps these can serve as a springboard for clinical creativity in readers.

Video Recording

As mentioned earlier, my working hypothesis about why posttraumatic play can become stuck is that children are not able to achieve a safe enough distance from the play. I have postulated that children's sensory involvement and externalizing in concrete form can be factors in their inability to establish or sustain required distance. Even when children are telling stories verbally or through action, with or without puppets in their fingers, they embody their story and thus remain connected to it in a powerful way—once again, the safe enough distance is not realized. Reflection is definitely a treatment goal, but it is more efficiently achieved through projection than through immediate ownership of feelings.

Once the recording is on a screen, children's attention can be directed to what they see rather than what they feel inside the play through physical contact. Video provides distance, and children may feel the safety they need.

Clinicians can subsequently give control of the video player to the child, allowing him or her to rewind, fast-forward, or pause. Clinicians can also then use some of the interventions mentioned earlier: narrative descriptions, voice-giving to characters, stopping and starting the play at different points and asking how characters think and feel throughout the play. In other words, clinicians introduce the kinds of activities and interactions that most children use when they are engaged in generic play therapy.

But using video can be complex. For example, children may have been abused, and a parallel legal process may be underway; it may therefore be counterindicated to make videos that could be subpoenaed. Some children may have been abused while others watched or recorded the abuse. Some children will cower at the idea of being filmed and may simply withdraw. I have found it important to explain to children that you are recording the play itself, not them. But for some children, recording is not possible or not desirable.

Reflective Mirrors

Another option that seemed effective on numerous occasions was to use a physical mirror so that children could focus on the reflection of the play. At times children have allowed me to record the reflections in the mirror, but nothing more. The basic goal of gaining some distance is met in this particular way, and there is an advantage to the transparency of the intervention (children can see what's going on) as well as the comfort in knowing that a permanent record of the play does not exist.

Story Boards

One effective idea is for clinicians to draw the narrative that the child has expressed in therapy. Putting the sequence of the story into graphic figures and reflecting back to children what they have shown so far can be useful. Some clinicians are reluctant to draw because they are unsure of their artistic ability. I once supervised an intern who solved this problem by doing a story board using cutouts from magazines and then narrating the picture to the child. When children engage with pictorial renditions of their traumatic stories, they may achieve the necessary distance for reflection. This method sometimes increases insight, understanding, or expression.

Once children achieve a safe distance in their play, they usually have varied responses: Sometimes they are truly able to reflect and allow themselves to be touched, moved, or inspired in some way. Their feelings can come to the surface, their perceptions can sharpen, and their thinking may clarify. This outcome of course depends on the age of the child and a number of other variables, including how much safety they have come to feel in the therapy relationship and how much support they have outside the therapy office. The purpose of these interventions is to create opportunities for the toxic play to shift toward a healthier and more positive outcome.

CONCLUSION

Posttraumatic play allows children to have a renewed sense of control and to gain mastery over traumatic memories. However, some children are not able to employ the dynamic aspects of posttraumatic play and instead find that this play gets stuck in negative outcomes.

I propose that children can be vulnerable to posttraumatic play because they may be so fully immersed in it that they do not achieve a safe enough distance. When children have experiences that are too painful or confusing, when they are consumed with fear or anxiety, when they are avoiding pain as best they can, when their brains are triggered to have responses that cause problem behaviors, then their natural reparative mechanisms might need assistance and facilitation to be wholly useful. In these situations, clinicians must respond to toxic posttraumatic play differently than they might respond to dynamic play that moves on its own toward resolution.

The continuum of interventions reviewed in this chapter ranges from less to more disruptive. They are designed to change the play's rigid status and to allow the release of a more useful energy. Some of these interventions are drawn directly from what play therapists know to be associated with healthy, generic play, and others are interventions that I've developed in response to my formulation of toxic posttraumatic play and my clinical experiences over the last four decades. They include video recording, the use of reflective mirrors, and the creation of story boards. Whether dynamic or toxic, posttraumatic play emerges in response to children's traumatic events and appears to provide a way for children to gain mastery over their prior experiences of helplessness and vulnerability.

4

Manifestations of Posttraumatic Play in Natural Settings and in the Therapy Office

*C*hildren can exhibit posttraumatic play in any setting eliciting interest and concern from others. This chapter discusses how posttraumatic play can become visible in a variety of ways in a variety of places. Its appearance is not limited to the clinical setting.

POSTTRAUMATIC PLAY IN SCHOOLS AND HOSPITALS

HOSPITAL

Four-year-old Miranda lived in a violent home in which her mother was regularly beaten by her father. She was taken to the hospital with peritonitis, had surgery for her burst appendix, and spent the next few days recovering. The nurses were fascinated to see that Miranda would often pound on her chest without any kind of provocation or apparent pain responses. In addition, she scratched herself, drawing blood, and she asked the nurses for Band-Aids to cover her hurts. When her mother visited, Miranda exhibited extreme ambivalent behaviors, sometimes stretching out her arms for hugs and other times hitting her playfully on the chest.

SCHOOL

Six-year-old Alex asked to go to the school nurse's office each afternoon without fail. There were no apparent medical concerns, but Alex was eager to have the nurse spend time with him. He kept insisting that he couldn't see very well, and the nurse would look deeply into his eyes. He then stated that he had a twitch, and the nurse would look at his eyes to ascertain whether twitching occurred. In addition, the child constantly talked about pain in his hands and encouraged the nurse to hold them, sometimes asking that they be rubbed.

HOSPITAL

Three-year-old Melinda was found alone in a filthy apartment. She had cockroaches in her ears that doctors removed. Her hair was matted, and maggots were thriving on her scalp. She had impetigo on her saddle area, and more than one laceration in her vaginal area. She had cigarette burns on her arms, and her ribs were protruding. She had obviously lived in dire circumstances with inconsistent and cruel caretaking. She had blisters in her mouth and barely muttered a sound when police picked her up and took her to the emergency room. She was severely dehydrated and was hospitalized for a few weeks prior to going to an emergency foster care placement. During her stay in the hospital, she preferred to be in her crib than out of it. She did not seek out attention from others. One of the nurses rocked her in a rocking chair for about 20 minutes every day. She became limp in the nurse's arms each time. By the end of the second week, Melinda would walk to the chair when the nurse came in. The hospital staff (nursing, social work, and psychiatry) was quite concerned with this child's developmental delays but became worried when Melinda kept stuffing her vagina full of gauze, toilet paper, or whatever else she could find.

SCHOOL

Nine-year-old Benjamin picked a fight almost every day at school. He was always sent to the principal's office where he would usually urinate into his pants. The principal would usually call his parents, and his mother would pick him up within an hour of receiving the call.

He had been expelled from three elementary schools, and his mother was frustrated and angered by his behaviors. Benjamin preferred to stay in his room and had developed a sudden anxious attachment to his parents, wanting to sleep with them and to be close to them throughout the day. His aggressive behaviors were new to his parents who thought it might be related to their recent marital conflicts.

All these situations involve children's behaviors in school or hospital settings, and they can cause confusion, baffling even the best trained professionals. These behaviors require that professionals consider them contextually, through the lens of possible trauma. A good rule of thumb is to view any confounding behavior as children's possible attempts at communication. Children in distress don't have typical mechanisms for expressing pain or asking for help. Instead, they find creative and age-appropriate ways to seek assistance. Below is my formulation of the behaviors described above as posttraumatic play or enactments.

• *Miranda.* I have always found it useful to try to "decode" children's behavior. This child had witnessed a great deal of abuse, so much so that the victim–victimizer dynamics had been well integrated into her understanding of the world and relationships between people. Upon further inquiry, I discovered that Miranda would usually consistently hit her chest when approached by a male nurse, who was very friendly with her. His overt friendliness created a great deal of anxiety in Miranda, who was unfamiliar with nice behavior in men. It was difficult for her to tolerate the anxiety she felt, so she hit herself instead. Miranda's behaviors, for example, can be viewed in at least two ways: (1) She is taking control of the situation by hurting herself so no one else can do it; and (2) her anxiety increases when she needs her mother, so she reenacts violence against women and girls, and in that way elicits mother's caretaking and limit-setting behaviors. I'm sure there are other interpretations of this behavior that could be posited. Miranda also scratched herself and bled. The nurses noticed that she wrote her name with the blood that she drew from her arms and stained her sheets. My understanding of this behavior was along the same lines as her beating herself. As she cut open her skin, she was deciding where the cuts would be made, how deeply, and how many.

It also became clear to me that for this child cutting served another purpose: As I got to know her in treatment, she described her "spacing-out" behaviors when her mother was being beaten. As she put it, "I just went away in my mind." It turned out that one of the ways that this child got deeper into her dissociative state was to cut. When I talked to Miranda's mother, I learned that Miranda's father had a cruel habit of putting hashtags on the mother's legs with a sharp knife when he was "a little bit mad at her." It's important to know that Miranda was referred to therapy by the hospital social worker who didn't understand Miranda's behavior but found it irregular enough to warrant a therapy referral. Miranda's mother, Sylvia, accepted the referral because she was "fed up" with her husband's behavior and could tell that it was affecting her daughter and her relationship with her daughter. The timing of this child's medical crisis facilitated a referral to mental health where the domestic violence was identified and services were provided to the mother to encourage her living in a safe family environment.

• *Alex* was living with a single father who worked three jobs. He was staying with multiple caretakers. Sometimes his father took him to work with him and left him to sleep in the truck until he was ready to go home. Alex's father, Jose, was a good, hard-working man whose wife Angela had died of cancer 3 years earlier. Jose and Angela had four other children in their country of origin, Nicaragua, and had planned for them to join them in the United States as soon as they were financially stable. When his wife died, Jose opted to keep his American-born son with him; they grieved together, and they vowed to make Angela's dreams for her children come true. So the father threw himself into working as much as he could. He never turned down a job. In the process, Alex got the short end of the stick. His father made sure he was well fed, had clean clothes, good shoes, and got to school on time. He was doing the very best he could and loved his son completely. However, he overlooked nurturing his child, holding him, kissing him, primping him, and showering him with the gazing, holding, and affection that Alex gravely missed. So Alex figured out a way to get some of his needs met: he would go to the nurse's office and force her to make eye contact with him, touch his face, and hold his hands. Eventually, this remarkable nurse understood this child's longing for physical touch and affection and referred the case to social services, who referred both father and son to treatment. They thrived in therapy, receiving a very structured, 3-month course of Theraplay (Booth & Jernberg, 2009), which was perfect for them.

• Fortunately, *Melinda* was identified after a neighbor called the police about a child believed to be alone in an apartment. When she was assessed in the emergency room, she was seen as a textbook example of a severely neglected child. She elicited warm and rigorous caretaking from staff in many departments of the hospital, and during her hospital stay she made many friends. One nurse, in particular, recognized Miranda's need for quiet, consistent, physical holding and provided that warmth to her daily, even returning on her day off to hold and rock the child in her arms. Melinda's body went limp when the nurse held her, but she eventually sought out the holding when the nurse came into the room. Melinda's initial responses were fear-based. Being held in a safe, nurturing manner was so unfamiliar to her that her brain sent alert messages to her body to go limp to keep her out of harm's way. The consistency of the nurse's daily caretaking allowed Melinda's brain to form new synapses and respond differently to physical touch, quieting the alarm signals and learning to trust.

The behavior that most mystified the hospital staff was Melinda's stuffing her vagina with whatever she could get her hands on. This turned out to be related to the extensive sexual abuse she had suffered. I view this behavior as posttraumatic behavior reenactment, as well as the child's way of calling attention to her particular situation and asking for help. A few possible reasons come to mind: First, she gains a sense of mastery: by filling her vaginal cavity, nothing else can enter. Only a traumatized child could imagine such an action, a simple and exquisite defense. A second interpretation might be simple reenactment in which she is showing anyone who will look her way the intrusion that she has experienced. Either scenario reflects a quality of resilience in Melinda, something remarkable and something growth-driven.

• *Benjamin's* situation was camouflaged by his aggression. His parents made the understandable error of assuming that the aggression and regressed behavior (bedwetting) were related to their recent marital problems. They confided that they were very close to divorcing and were concerned about their only son. They were eager to have him in therapy and were surprised when they were asked to participate in the treatment.

The initial therapy phase went smoothly, but Benjamin appeared hypervigilant and unusually skittish for a 9-year-old boy. He did not exhibit defiance or anger in the therapy office; instead he responded in a compliant way that stood out as unusual. We made cautious progress, and when I invited his parents into the session, his anxious attachment was obvious. His parents insisted that this was new behavior and they didn't like it because he was acting so much younger and less mature than they knew him to be.

I continued to work with Benjamin individually for a few more months, and finally, he took to the sand tray and built a very long, snake-like mound in the sand. At the end of this snake, he made a face and attempted to use construction paper to make a snake's tongue, but the tongue turned into something else, something that looked like an "8." He then colored in the number and put it over a yellow piece of construction paper and cut it out. Now it looked like the snake was leaking urine or peeing in the tray. He volunteered that it was a snake, "a really long, mean snake." When I asked him to tell me more about the snake, he said, "That's it. He's mean." I pointed to the yellow shape coming out of his mouth and said I noticed how carefully he had made it, having cut it out twice, once in green and once in yellow. When he did not volunteer any answer, I asked him what it was. "I wonder what that could be?" I hesitated and then I said, "Is he peeing?" "No," he said loudly, "if he was peeing, it would be coming out of his pee hole." "Oh," I said, "you're right, this is coming out of his mouth." "Right!" he said. Before I could say anything else, he said, "I'm gonna kill him with my bare hands." He proceeded to pound on his snake until it was completely destroyed. "I'm stronger than I look," he said as he finished what he was doing. In the following session, he made the same shape again and pounded it over and over. This play seemed intense and focused. By the fourth session, I made another guess. "I've been thinking if maybe that's vomit coming out of his mouth." "No," Ben said, "but you're getting closer." Within a few more weeks he was able to tell me that it was "sticky white stuff" that came out of "other places." That led us to talk about penises and ejaculation, and he confided that a male teenage babysitter had forced him to perform fellatio. Benjamin was compelling as he described not being able to get this picture out of his mind, even though he never saw this babysitter again and he never said anything to his parents. The combination of wetting himself and beating on others was precisely embedded in his play and indicative of unresolved traumatic material, silently held in his mind. His thoughts and feelings were overwhelming to him, and even worse for this child was his self-imposed isolation. When he finally allowed me to tell his parents about what had happened to him, he wept in his parents' arms for a full hour.

When traumatic incidents occur to young children, the impact can range from minor to extensive. What we know for sure is that children endeavor to manage their stress and fears, and they make numerous efforts to communicate their distress to those around them. Thus, posttraumatic play or behaviors can be observed in multiple settings, especially schools and hospitals. It's important to decode children's behaviors keeping in mind the possibility of childhood trauma.

POSTTRAUMATIC PLAY IN THE THERAPY OFFICE

I encourage clinical attention to signs of posttraumatic play no matter what form it takes. Because of its name, some clinicians assume that posttraumatic play exists only in traditional play activities. In fact, posttraumatic play surfaces in art creations, in sand tray scenarios, in stories, in miniature work, and in children's behaviors and interactions with others. Clinicians are thus advised to develop strategies to identify, discern, and accommodate children's posttraumatic play in the clinical setting.

LIZZIE: AN EXAMPLE OF THERAPEUTIC ART

Lizzie was a 12-year-old who had lived in six foster homes, while her mother, Stephanie, attempted and failed numerous drug counseling programs before leaving town for good. Lizzie had lived in a foster-adopt home for approximately 2 years and for the most part, had done fairly well adapting to a family with older children in college. For all intents and purposes, her foster mother, Dora, had made a significant investment in Lizzie's well-being. She was a patient and kind woman whose husband had died from a sudden heart attack when her college children were in elementary school. At this time of her life, Dora wanted to commit to the long-term care of another child and cherished her role as a parent.

Lizzie was a bright, attractive, and compliant child. She had not exhibited any acting-out behavior until she heard that her mother's parental rights were going to be terminated. Throughout her long stay in foster care with Dora, her mother's visits had been erratic and Lizzie had developed a way of coping that included acting detached. At one of our sessions she confided, "I don't like to wait for things to happen; if they happen great, if not, I don't care." Clearly, she had learned to lower her expectations to avoid feeling gravely disappointed.

Most professionals felt this adoption was a given; they could not foresee the acute episode that brought this family to a crisis and caused everyone to reconsider Lizzie's placement with Dora.

The first event occurred when Lizzie regressed profoundly, defecating in several rooms of the house, cutting Dora's clothes, setting a small fire that burned her mattress, and generally decompensating to the extent that she was hospitalized. She was hospitalized for two weeks, and once stabilized, she was referred to me for play therapy since she was unable or unwilling to articulate her experience verbally. The precipitating factor had likely been Lizzie's being told by her caseworker that her mother's parental rights would be terminated. Dora was quite confused by Lizzie's behavior. She was adamant that she didn't want to do anything that could make Lizzie unhappy or uncomfortable.

Treatment began smoothly. I set the context for therapy by explaining what I knew about her recent difficulties. Dora stayed in the room for about 15 minutes and then intuitively knew to leave. Lizzie was shy and well behaved, and she explored the room with great hesitation. She zeroed in on a Baby Alive doll that drank a bottle and then urinated. Lizzie asked if there were clothes and blankets and diapers, and I pulled out what was available. She set them aside in the first session but played with them with abandon in subsequent sessions.

Her favorite routine was to feed the baby and allow her to pee. She then undressed her, bathed her, washed her hair, and dried and combed it. She seemed happy doing this over and over; clearly, this play helped her process something important.

About 2 months of this play was followed by a change in the routine. At this juncture, Lizzie asked for paints and decided she wanted to paint on large pieces of easel paper. She made circles, filling them with different colors, and seemed absorbed with this experience. She left each session happy, and Dora noted that her behaviors at home had returned to usual. I surmised that Lizzie had compartmentalized her feelings about her mother and would not likely have another episode unless the topic was raised again.

I let her paint for two sessions without interruption. She then told me that she would be making a painting of flowers. She said that she would sketch it out first to make sure it came out perfectly. She seemed enthusiastic about this project and became highly focused on it. It was gratifying to see her invest herself so completely, and although I did not know exactly what the content of the picture would be, it was clear that she was preparing for creative self-expression.

The first line drawing appeared innocuous and simple: Three large flowers that emerged from grass on the bottom of the page. The flowers appeared to be daisies and the petals were ample. As this sketch evolved, it was clear that there were two large flowers on the left and right and a smaller one in the middle. Lizzie was very careful as she began to paint them, and she went to great lengths to keep her painting inside the firm boundaries she had drawn.

The small flower in the center of the painting captured her attention and time. The inside of the flower was black and the outside petals were bright pink. The flower on the left was reversed in color schemes, with a bright pink center and black petals. Finally, the flower on the right had an orange and pink center and the petals alternated between purple, blue, and red. This was indeed the brightest flower in the picture. When she finished the picture, she sat back and said, "How come my mom doesn't want me?" I remarked that this was a big question and wondered what she thought the answer would be if she asked her mom. "I don't know," she said. Then she added, "My mom likes drugs more than me." "Oh," I said, "so you're thinking that your mom chooses to do drugs instead of take care of you." She nodded her head. I told her I could understand her feeling that way. I resisted the urge to use psychoeducation at this moment since Lizzie seemed to have tears in her eyes as she held her wet paintbrush. I simply put my arm around her shoulder and said, "It sounds like your mom is on your mind." She wiped away her tears and added, "Just sometimes I wonder what was wrong with me that she doesn't want me." Again, I simply stroked her back a little and noted that I could see how she might think that. I then asked her how that made her feel. "Sad," she said, "and mad!" I reassured her that it was okay to feel whatever feelings she felt toward her mom and that her relationship to her had for certain been quite difficult. We were quiet the rest of the time, and as she left, I told her that anytime she wanted to talk more or show me anything about her mom, I was ready to listen. I also told her that it might be good to talk about what to do about her feelings of sadness and anger. At that, she seemed to leave more abruptly than at other times.

When Lizzie returned for the next session, she quickly returned to her routine, telling me that "I don't want to talk today." I told her that was fine and that she could choose how to spend her time. In this session, she returned to her painting, touching up everything she could, reaffirming some of the lines, and thinking about the background and what color she wanted to use.

As Lizzie kept painting I noticed that the left flower had a great deal of black and had a different feel and energy than the flower on the right side, opposite her. Every little subtle change that she made seemed to be well thought out. As she had done in a previous session, she would often stop and gaze at her picture, looking far away in silence.

The painting was finally finished, and I pulled up a chair and asked that we look at it together. I told her she could say as much or as little as she wanted. She shrugged her shoulder. I asserted that she had made this painting very carefully and with great purpose. I wondered how she felt when she looked at the final product. Again she didn't respond. She told me to keep the painting in the office until the following week when she might take it home. I secretly thought of buying a frame for it, to honor what she had done in a concrete way. On the way out, I had an idea that I shared impulsively: "Do me a favor," I said to Lizzie. "Before you go to sleep tonight, write a letter from the small flower to the big ones. Pick who you would like to write to first and then second. Good luck."

She returned to therapy and opted to retouch her painting. She did this the following five sessions, and as she did, she spoke in a hushed and consistent tone. She created a solemn mood as she spoke first in random sentences and later began to use complete, coherent sentences. During this time I sat next to her, slightly behind her, and maintained the silence she seemed to demand. As I was silent, there was room for her to come forward. The following major themes were revealed (although I'm uncertain of the order):

She chose to write a letter to the flower on her left, the one with the black petals. She retouched the black as she spoke with very soft, barely detectable strokes. "Black petals are pretty." "Sometimes plants turn black because they don't get watered." "Winter kills." "Sometimes they grow back different colors." "I like black petals." "Petals are meant to be pretty colors . . . black is pretty." I had countless interpretations of what she was saying, but it soon became evident that in her trance-like free association she was addressing compelling issues about her mother, her mother's history and lack of nurturing, how change was possible, and how, even though black is not a typical color for flowers, it was nevertheless a pretty color that she herself liked. It seemed that she was trying to negotiate her feelings about her mother being different, unique, offputting, and possibly still an attachment figure to her, in spite of her minimal presence in her life. The metaphor she used in this painting seemed to symbolize this child's longing for her mother and the crisis that had ensued after she discovered her mother's more permanent absence from her life.

The painting was almost like a love letter to her mother as well as representing her permanent connection to her mother. The reversed colors were an example of this sentiment, as was the sharing of a small piece of land in which the three flowers grew. Her painting also seemed to demonstrate her turning toward her new attachment figure, Dora, and her ability to shift away from her mother to more fully embrace her permanent placement with Dora. Lizzie eventually invited her foster mother into the session to "pick up" her painting. She wanted the three of us to sit in front of the easel. Lizzie told Dora to "pull up a chair so that we can look at this together." Dora complied and listened as Lizzie explained that the flower on the left was her mother who had "birthed" her and the flower on the right was Dora, who would be taking over for her first mother. At some point, Lizzie sat on Dora's lap and played with her hair like a much younger child would, and together they decided where in the house they would hang this very important, lovely painting that had allowed Lizzie to face her traumatic loss in her unique way.

DEREK: AN EXAMPLE OF PLAY THERAPY

Six-year-old Derek had recently learned that his parents would be getting divorced. He had a very acute response—he ran up to his room, locked the door, and wouldn't come out for hours. He sobbed loudly as both of his parents sat outside the room until his father said he was leaving. At that point Derek came out and kicked his dad, spit at his mother, and screamed loudly and relentlessly—so much so that the neighbors came over to make sure that everything was all right, which quieted him down for a little while. His father's bags were packed, and he left that night for a new apartment about two hours away. Derek's mother had wanted to break the news to him in a different way, but being distressed and worried, she had not crafted a better plan. Everything moved quickly after the announcement, and the father moved out. Derek's mother returned to her former job, Derek was supervised by a childcare worker after school, and their home was put on the market. Derek's primary mode of expression was anger, and he kicked, shoved, yelled, and frequently threw things at his mother. During the first 2 months of the separation, Derek saw his father twice, partly because his father was still getting his apartment ready and partly because his new promotion at work required that he put in long hours.

I saw Derek in the third month after his parent announced their separation. He was unhappy about coming to therapy, although the toys in the office clearly soothed his fighting spirit. He spent the first two sessions exploring the room, taking things out of their cabinets, spreading things about, and going from one item to another. In the first session, when I asked why he was coming to see me, he said, "I don't care." When I asked if he knew why, he simply shrugged. I told him that his mother had told me that she and Derek's dad were getting a divorce and that Derek was pretty darn angry about that. He looked at me when I said that, and I added: "You have every right to feel some anger. Divorce stinks!" He walked away and began to look around.

Every now and then it appeared that Derek wanted to live up to the reputation that his frustrated and quite verbal mother had so vividly described to me. Every session she wanted to spend the first 10 minutes or so telling me all the things Derek had done that were destructive, annoying, or both. I thereupon sent her an email asking her to fill out a one-page series of questions so that I could read it before the sessions started. The questions were: "What delighted you about your son this week? Can you tell me a happy surprise you had with him? Can you list three things that show that he's improving on those behaviors that concern you?" The last question was: "Do you have any current concerns about Derek's behaviors?" The mother complied with my request and was able to start identifying some positives with Derek, but she always expounded on the last question. It was painfully clear that Derek's mother was struggling and that she felt abandoned to care for her angry child. What distressed her even more was that Derek began to behave in a compliant manner with his father, who as a result continually accused her of not knowing how to handle him.

I requested that the mother meet with one of our therapists while she waited for Derek's therapy appointment. She agreed to talk to someone, although she asked for someone who was older and perhaps had children and had gone through a divorce. We were able to satisfy those requests, and she quickly found herself feeling more competent about how to handle her son. The collateral therapy with the mother was very helpful to Derek's treatment. As for Derek's father, he repeatedly stated that he was too busy to come into therapy and that Derek was "doing just fine."

Derek was a strong-willed child, bright and creative, and he loved to laugh. He also clearly manipulated situations to meet his needs, cheated shamefully at games, and was acutely ambivalent about expressing his feelings verbally. I used a number of expressive techniques that helped him identify and show his feelings about things. The Color Your Feelings technique (Hopkins, Huici, & Bermudez, 2005), in particular, gave him a chance to show how he felt when his dad lived in the house and now that dad lived in his own apartment.

It was interesting to see that the drawings were compatible and that the before and after feelings were almost indistinguishable. When I pointed out how similar his paintings were, he threw them first on the ground and then in the sand. Over time, a more complete picture of family dynamics developed, and it became apparent that the divorce had not been a surprise to this child. It turned out that his parents had slept in different rooms for almost a year, that they used the "silent treatment" when they were angry at each other, and that the father spent most of his waking hours at a very demanding and competitive job. Both parents confirmed all these facts and asserted that they should have divorced years ago.

Any attempts to talk to Derek about the divorce directly were not useful. But he found some creative ways to bring the issue of divorce into the clinical setting. Derek had explored the dollhouse on numerous occasions, sometimes clearing out all the furniture and throwing it on the ground, other times, moving things around. One day, I purposely left two adult figures and one child in the dollhouse, and I made sure they resembled Derek and his parents: the boy was brown-haired like Derek was, the mother blonde, and the father brown-haired, and both were younger looking. I made a big fuss that someone had left toys in the dollhouse without putting them away. I told him that I felt anger when people don't clean up after themselves. "Look at this," I stated. "Someone has left a dad, mom, and kid in the dollhouse!" I started to pick them up. "Wait," Derek said, "Let me look." He took each of the dolls and looked at them and then he said, "That's okay, they can stay." I said "okay." Later in the session, he asked if I had rubber bands. "Oh," I said, "I don't have any with me. I do have some, just somewhere else." Then he asked if I had scotch tape that I could provide. He took the scotch tape and put the two dolls facing each other and started putting pieces of scotch tape, one after the other, until he had in essence bound the mother and father figures together. He showed them to me with pride, "NOW they have to stay together in the house." I agreed and they were placed back. I asked if he still wanted rubber bands; he replied yes, and so I offered to bring them next time. When he put the taped adults in the dollhouse, he placed them in the big double bed and said, "They better be there when I get back!" "Well," I said, "you know how that goes, people should put things back when they use the toys in this room." "Okay," he negotiated, "then let's just hide them so no one sees them." He took the bed with the two taped dolls and found an excellent hiding place. "No one will find them here." He was right, no one did!

The following week he was very excited to see that his taped masterpiece was still in its place. He was also excited about the ball of rubber bands I had brought in for him. I do not exaggerate when I say that he spent the whole session putting rubber bands around the couple until it appeared round. My job was to pass him the rubber bands, and his job was to put them around the couple until he formed a rather large ball. He completed this project at the next session and then he said, "Okay, let's play catch." What began as a simple game of catch turned into something quite intense as he started throwing the rubber ball into the walls, so much so that I had to move the throwing session outside so he could use the outside wall. His energy intensified as he threw the ball over and over until he fell to the ground fatigued. "I hate him," he exclaimed. "Who's him?" I asked. "My dad! I hate him!" I told him that sometimes we have strong feelings about people we love. "I don't love him, I hate him!" When I asked what he hated the most, he answered, "that he moved far away from us." I sat with him and said I was sorry that he felt badly about his parents. "They're supposed to stay married," he screamed. "I know," I repeated, "parents are supposed to stay married. When they don't, it's hard on the kids." Quite unexpectedly he jumped into my arms; I held him and told him I was sorry.

TAMMY: AN EXAMPLE OF SAND THERAPY

Seven-year-old Tammy's father had recently been injured while deployed with the Air Force. Her mother had been working as an elementary school teacher. Tammy had a brother, Michael, 12, as well as a sister Gracie, 2 years older than she was. Tammy's mother had become very depressed with her husband's five consecutive deployments, In the past year, she had asked her mother, Tammy's grandmother, to take care of the two older children. Tammy had been born prematurely, and so her mother had been very protective of her since the time she was born. Tammy had been a good student, but the teachers called home when they noticed that Tammy seemed worried, despondent, and inattentive in the classroom. Concerned about her sudden changes in behavior, they encouraged Tammy's mother to take her to a counselor. The mother was compliant, especially since she was feeling depressed and guilty about her lack of energy and inattention to her children.

During the intake session, the mother's depression was obvious in her flat, monotonous presentation. She wiped away her tears carefully and spoke softly. She described her current level of inactivity, lethargy, and lack of motivation. I gave her a lot of encouragement for "dragging" herself out of bed to go to work each day. She commented that with three children she needed to bring in extra income while her husband was away. She described her husband as a "career person" with the Air Force and talked about his many deployments. I inquired if she had social support from other spouses or partners of Air Force personnel. She said that she knew quite a few wives in the area but didn't feel she had time to be in touch with them. "I think I said no to so many invitations, they don't call me anymore." She said she had been to the Air Force's DFS in the past but felt ashamed to return yet again. "I shouldn't be asking for help; I'm one of the lucky ones. My husband is home now, and even though he's injured, he will get better." She knocked on wood, and I commented that I was happy that her husband's injuries would heal. But I also told her that I was concerned that she felt she could not avail herself of resources because she assumed that her counselors would judge her for seeking them out "yet again." I asked her to think about getting counseling for herself while her daughter was in treatment, but she answered that there wasn't enough time in the day. Given how she responded, I told her I was impressed with her making time for her daughter and I would see if we could meet from time to time to check on how she was doing and to keep her informed of her daughter's progress. When I asked how her husband felt about Tammy coming to therapy, she said: "We both feel that she really needs the help. I can tell, we both can, that something's off with her." She didn't offer too many of her own concerns, instead saying that she trusted the teachers and believed that her daughter was experiencing distress.

When I met with Tammy, I found her to be a sweet, compliant child, somewhat small for her age. She looked up at me a lot, waiting for cues as to what to do next or what to say. I tried to get her to explore the playroom, but she kept asking for directives. A few times when she took out a toy, she put it back carefully and thanked me for letting her play with it. She seemed very curious about the sandbox but was initially reluctant to go near it. She finally put her finger in tentatively and made a little hole that she covered up quickly. I put my hand into the tray and moved the sand around freely, modeling that she did not need to be so careful. It took about four sessions for her to feel comfortable enough to choose her own activities. She seemed most interested in the sandbox, and although she put her fingers in the tray every time she saw me, on this one occasion, she asked if she could put some things inside the tray. She brought over two ponies and laid them down, covering them with sand carefully. She also brought over a bull and placed him in the corner of the tray, far away from the ponies, and covered it up with sand. She then took a mother and baby lamb and placed them in yet another part of the tray, covering them up as well. She patted the sand so that you really couldn't tell where the animals were buried. She took a car and moved it around the sand tray, but it appeared as if the car never ran over the buried animals in the tray. Her tone was hushed as she did this, and when I remarked that there were two lambs, two ponies, and one bull, she simply nodded in affirmation. I noted that they were in different places and she nodded her head again. After this first time of playing with these five objects, I noted that there were a total of five animals, one of which was alone and the others in two's. She shook the sand off her hands and left with a little smile on her face. She didn't ask whether they would be there when she returned, nor did she ask if she should return them to their proper place, common questions from children who use the sand tray for the first time.

The following six sessions were a repetition of the scenario Tammy had created with the five objects. Each time there was the same hushed tone. The child sat back in her chair, caressing the objects prior to placing them in the sand and using for about the same amount of time. The play was rote and rigid, and Tammy never varied her approach. At about the third session, I said, "I wonder what it's like for the bull to be by himself?" She sat back in her chair, went to the corner, pulled out the bull, and replaced him in the same spot. She didn't respond to me and didn't like talking to me while she worked. When she was in the room with the sand tray, she did not speak much at all. When we walked out of the play therapy office into a smaller office with chairs and a couch, she would sometimes climb onto the couch and ask questions about different things. One day she said, "Do you see other kids whose dads are in the army?" "Yes," I told her, "I see some kids whose dads or moms are in the army." "Moms fight in the war?" she asked incredulous. "Yes," I said, "some moms also work in the army." When the session was over, she straight-away ran out to announce this fact to her mother. Another time she asked if I had grandkids, and I told her I did. She asked their ages and I told her. She told me her grandmother lived far away. When I asked if she visited her, she said, "Not right now. She's busy." When I asked what kept her busy, she got off the couch and said it was time to go. Her reluctance to volunteer any personal information seemed different to me, and yet her play seemed to present some of her family dynamics: The two ponies were likely her older siblings, the two lambs were likely herself and her mother (she said big one and little one), and the bull, who was most removed, could have been her dad. My working hypothesis was that the separation from her father and siblings had left her in a close bind with her mother, who was often depressed, unavailable, and fragile. This little girl likely saw herself as her mother's caretaker while her father was away, and her siblings were not around to help.

This hypothesis grew more relevant as Tammy's play proceeded and her periods of gazing from the chair became longer. There was an emotional distance in this child that seemed unusual. At about session 8, she was gazing at the hidden figures, and I wondered out loud whether the figures knew that the others were nearby even if they couldn't see them. She didn't respond at first, and then she began placing some rocks between them, creating what appeared to be paths on top of the sand. When she left the session, she left the rocks in place, asking me to make sure no one would take them.

These paths became more elaborate with smaller pebbles. She also put down some bridges, some fences, and some trees. The trays appeared to have a little more energy (movement between objects and her investment in the creation), and she would get out from her chair, look around at the miniatures, and place more and more objects in the tray. I then commented on how there was something going on underneath the sand and on top of the sand. At that session, she went to each of her little hidden objects and, using a brush, cleared away enough sand to see a little tiny bit of each object. Finally, they were slightly visible.

As the tray took on a different look, she became slightly more engaged with me. Sometimes, instead of moving to the other room to talk from the couch, she would wander around the room and talk to me about different things.

At about session 13, the objects came to the surface after being buried for just a brief time. "Oh," I noted, "they have come into the light. I wonder what they see." "Each other," she said matter of factly. "And how do they feel about seeing each other?" I asked. "They don't know," she said, "it's been a long time." "Oh," I repeated, "so they don't know what they think or feel about seeing each other again." "Shy," she said, "they don't look the same." At that point, she wondered into the other room, and when I followed she asked me if my dad lived with me. "Not now," I said, "when I was little he did." "Is he dead now?" she asked, and I said "Yes." "My dad almost died," she told me. "Oh, I didn't know that." "My mom thought he was going to come back in a box with a flag on it." "Oh, so your mom was worried about your dad when he was away." "And me too!" she said, "I worry he's still going to die and my mom too!"

She went out the door, and I was happy that she was finally speaking about the things that she had carried around in her head. I noticed that she was struggling to release this information and that she avoided contact with me whenever she said something momentous to herself. I made a mental note to meet with her parents and discuss how they could support her given the amazing stress she had endured. I also wondered about her siblings and when they would be returning home as well as what they had told Tammy about why they left.

I first met with the parents alone, and later I met with the family. During the parents' meeting, we talked about some of my observations and concerns. I started out by saying that children take in a lot of stressful information these days about the war, safety, and danger, and about a lot of other family things. I also told them that children are uniquely focused on their parents and on making sure they are happy and safe. I noted that Tammy had had a lot of stressors in the past year: her father's deployments and being in harm's way, her separation from her siblings, and her mother's depression. I told the parents that I believed it would be critical to their daughter's mental health to speak directly and clearly to her and to articulate what had been happening to the family. I also noted that it seemed to me that their family had a habit of avoidance when dealing (or not dealing) with stressors, a particular habit that is counterproductive. It can contribute to a host of unexpressed feelings. The parents were receptive to my feedback, and a number of family therapy sessions ensued, designed to create nurturing, empathic interactions between Tammy and her parents and to provide accurate information about her father's job status (he would not be deployed again), her mother's improving depression, and why her siblings were sent away (the mother felt she was unable to take care of them). Tammy also asked many questions, including why her mother was sad all the time. Most importantly, she wanted to know when her siblings would come home. Tammy also wondered if her dad liked living away from home. All these substantive and confusing issues were clarified, and Tammy benefited greatly from discussing them. Six months later when her siblings returned, Tammy asked her mother if they could come see her "special play place," and I was happy to oblige.

RAUL: AN EXAMPLE OF MINIATURE WORK

Paul was a 12-year-old who was referred to therapy after witnessing his older brother's shooting death. Paul, his brother, and his family lived in a high-risk, low-income neighborhood with their single mother who worked two jobs to keep her head above water financially. Paul's 19-year-old brother, Sam, had been recruited into a gang at about 10 years of age and had recently gotten out. Unfortunately, his attempts to extricate himself ended up in violence and tragedy. Paul was left with a range of intense and difficult emotions. Paul and Sam were very close, with Sam serving in a parental role to his younger brother. Paul's mother tried her best to comfort her young son after his brother's death, but Paul was inconsolable and began to behave in an extremely impulsive way.

At school Paul would initiate fights at recess. He was provocative with his peers, for example, throwing rocks or dirt at them. He used inflammatory language and constantly made threats. Half the time he hurt others, and half the time he hurt himself. All his interactions were directed at older or bigger boys, and there was no apparent explanation for his violent interactions. His teacher was very empathetic toward him and knew about his brother's murder, so she gave him every possible chance to calm down. But Paul was driven by rage and profound feelings of helplessness. He was mad at the world, could not be consoled, and was filled with intense emotions of anger, sadness, and fear.

After one of his suspensions, the school principal told Paul's mother that she had to get therapy for him before he would readmit Paul to school. Under pressure, his mother contacted her cousin whose son had also been in therapy, though for very different reasons. The mother thus contacted our office asking for help for her son. After meeting with her, I opted to refer her son to a male therapist whom I supervised. They met, and the mother was filled with confidence. I worked closely with my supervisee on this case; his posttraumatic play is chronicled here.

Paul was loath to attend therapy, as his behavior clearly communicated. He spat, pushed, and generally dismantled the therapy office. My intern, David, was committed to being patient, calm, and consistent with his demeanor, to maintaining rules, and to accepting Paul's self-expression as long as it wasn't a danger to himself or others. Paul pushed the limits as far as he could, one day swinging his arm around in such a way that it hit David in the nose and he began to bleed profusely. Paul, expecting to get in trouble, ran out of the room and into the waiting room. David followed with handkerchief in hand and told Paul that he would see him next week. When the person transporting Paul asked what happened, David simply said, "Just an accident, nothing to worry about." That inattention to the accident may have had an impact on Paul because the following week his behavior seemed less chaotic. Each week it was a step forward and three steps backwards until Paul began a very rigid routine in his play: He would enter the room, kick over the trash can, get a dinosaur puppet, and stuff its mouth with smaller puppets, especially a ladybug, a mouse, and a small deer. "I'm going to shove these down your throat until you throw up blood!" Then he would have the puppet throw up, and he would slap the puppet over and over. "Now you've done it, you poor excuse for a person, now you're gonna clean up all this mess or else!!!" The three small puppets would run away and get under the overturned trashcan so that they would be completely hidden. "If I find your ass, it's going to be grass under my lawnmower!!!" After this, Paul wanted to run outside and opened the door and took off quickly; David learned to follow with speed, concerned that Paul would run into the parking lot. Later, Paul and David developed a series of physical games that involved catch. Paul had a great left hand and could throw a ball with precision and speed. David would catch it and encourage him to throw it high, so that they both ran for the catch.

Paul's routine persisted for months. In time, David's check-in with the school and Paul's mother both began to sound promising: Paul's violent behavior was showing signs of decreasing in both frequency and intensity. David trusted that something important was going on in therapy and was convinced of this fact when the puppet play shifted to include the presence of a "fierce lion" who stopped the shoving of the smaller puppets into the others' mouths. The lion roared and shook wildly until the puppet let go of the small puppets, and then the lion took them one by one to the corner of the room. When they were in the corner, Paul put a blanket over them so that no one could see them. The lion then hushed them and told them that no one would hurt them again. It was clear that the lion was Paul's brother, who had rescued and protected him over and over again in the past. Over time, the lion then proceeded to do many other things in the room until the play ended, and Paul became much more interested in dyadic interventions with David.

CONCLUSION

Children's posttraumatic play can become noticeable in the clinical setting as well as in their natural environments such as home or school. Posttraumatic play is often dramatic and compelling, but at other times it is disguised, quiet, and overlooked. Clinicians need to be attentive to the emergence of this play and to be prepared to invite and facilitate clinical processing.

5

The Larger Treatment Context

A Systemic Approach to Posttraumatic Play

*T*he support, reassurance, guidance, and nurturance of (non-offending) parents of sexually abused children are necessary components of healing. The emergence or continuation of children's symptomatic behavior can be correlated to the type and extent of parental support and overall functioning in both Type I (Silverman & La Greca, 2002; Vernberg, 2002) and Type II traumas (Cohen & Mannarino, 1998; Lanktree & Briere, 2017). Complex trauma, in particular, may include a family system in which attachment is compromised and parenting may be inconsistent or neglectful (Blaustein & Kinniburgh, 2010). The growing literature claims that the recovery environment, and especially parental functioning, are much more significant for a child's posttraumatic adaptation than are the characteristics of the event itself (Cohen, 2009).

The importance of parental involvement cannot be overstated. The need for parental support makes absolute sense given that children take their cues from their parents. When stressful, harmful, confusing, or traumatic events occur, children need parental reassurance that things will be restored to normalcy. Younger children will require consistent comfort and reassurance from available parents. Older children are likewise dependent on parents to anchor themselves after difficult experiences. Thus, strengthening parental capacities, especially those related to nurturing, empathic interactions, is of great significance.

No other situation could be more destabilizing than an interpersonal traumatic experience (or in complex trauma, repeated experiences) in which children are left feeling helpless, confused, and vulnerable—longing for safety, direction, and encouragement. Children will almost always recover more easily if they have a guiding hand from a trusted parent or other caretaker.

Too often, parent–child dyadic work is not a required intervention. The most typical services provided to parents consist of giving them written or verbal psychoeducation alone or in groups, and encouraging them to provide sensitive, appropriate, and trauma-informed approaches to their children. There appears to be an overreliance on this type of approach as opposed to working with parent–child dyads or providing family therapy. Little assurance is given that the material provided to parents is ever fully understood or implemented in the long term, even though these efforts are critical to restored or improved family relationships. I have found and utilized several recent theoretical approaches that include psychoeducation in an accessible and practical way (Blaustein & Kinniburgh, 2010; Siegel & Bryson, 2011).

Lieberman and van Horn (2004b) developed an evidence-based therapy program for children who had witnessed domestic violence. They incorporated a focus on parent–child dyads guiding them to play together and using a psychoanalytic approach in which they used interpretation. This program thereby makes direct attempts to restore the parent to a position of authority and nurturance. Lieberman and van Horn noted that in many cases of domestic violence, the child was affected by experiencing their parent as another victim—maternal victimization often interfered with maternal protection of the children (see, e.g., Chapters 6 and 14 of the present volume).

In cases of childhood trauma, it is important to restore the parent's role as a trusted adult, capable of protecting the children. This enhances attachment and can change the child's internal working model—the child's view of the world and the people in it.

Another evidence-based program is parent–child interaction therapy for working with Type II traumas, specifically physically abused and neglected children (Eyberg, 1988). Other promising dyadic therapies that value play therapy as one of the healing factors include filial therapy (the original family therapy that promoted work with young children and their parents; Guerney, 2000; Van-Fleet, 2013) as well as child–parent relationship therapy (Bratton, Landreth, Kellam, & Blackard, 2006). Both of these models have great applicability to work with traumatized children, although neither is primarily recognized for that population.

Another well-established dyadic therapy that we have fully integrated into our trauma-focused treatment program at the Gil Institute is Theraplay. It is unique in strengthening or establishing attachment patterns (Booth & Jernberg, 2009).

This chapter discusses utilizing posttraumatic play within the context of family work with children and broader therapy services. My basic premise is that children need real opportunities to employ posttraumatic play on their own. Once this occurs, it is in the child's best interest for primary caretakers to help their children share narratives and thereby give them closure. Clinicians are well advised to assess parental capacities to provide empathic and child-centered responses. Parents' receptivity to therapeutic guidance and their emotional investment in their children are critical factors associated with positive treatment outcomes. The case illustrations that follow in Chapters 6 through 13 present a wide continuum of parental responses and capacities to put children's needs in front of their own.

I have found the following approaches important to the systemic treatment of childhood trauma.

INDIVIDUAL THERAPY WITH CHILDREN

Children need an opportunity to do some initial work on their own—a place unencumbered by adult expectations or demands. Professionals then need to gauge the parents' abilities to provide helpful responses to children. The parents or caretakers who join their children in family therapy are generally motivated to help their children and have demonstrated that they can provide safe and appropriate interactions with their children. Too often, however, parents who bring children to therapy have their own ideas about their children's needs and may convey these wishes, fears, and hopes directly or indirectly. The reality is that many parents are often on a different time clock about recovery than their children are. Their anxiety can be palpable to young children, who are used to discerning parents' mood states, desires, or concerns. Thus, children of anxious parents can develop their own set of anxieties (Wilson & Lyons, 2013). Caring parents may feel desperate to get a better understanding, to help their children immediately, to know what's going on deep in the recesses of their children's minds. Sometimes they want children to "get over" their abuse quickly and completely—helping children forget what happened is one of the most consistent requests that parents make of clinicians. Children and therapists alike can feel parental pressure whether or not it is spoken. Parents typically believe that they keep their sadness or worry hidden from their children, and yet children are known to do great detective work within their families.

I have provided therapy to children who are greatly inhibited by having parents in the room. It has nothing to do with what the parents are doing consciously. It has to do with children checking in constantly to see how their parents feel about what they say and do. Sometimes parents are unaware of how they are communicating nonverbally; they feel that as long as they are not saying anything directly to the child, they are not influencing them. Too often a parent who says "I promise to be out of your way" is a looming presence sitting in the corner. Parents can convey anxiety, expectations or demands, fears and worry in their tone of voice, their physical posture, and in physical signs of distress. Children are great at reading their parents' clues; they often know how their parents feel before the parents themselves know. Sometimes parents cannot control their responses. They may have their own memories of childhood trauma that surface at the very moment their children need their help most. For all these reasons, it's important for children to have a chance to express themselves alone for a period of time.

PARALLEL WORK FOR PARENTS

In my experience, children's traumatic experiences can put into motion a broad range of parental and familial reactions, questions, and concerns. One of the most concerning, and yet common, parental issues has already been mentioned: parental history of trauma. Some parents have conscious memories of abuse and have spent a great deal of energy in an overprotective stance. In some cases, protectiveness has been their single organizing focus as parents. They feel devastated that their substantive efforts to protect their children have failed. They may feel overwhelming guilt and fear that they will not be able to protect them in the future.

For other parents, the opposite is true. They may have compartmentalized and sealed off their own histories of abuse in an attempt to avoid pain or discomfort. When their children are abused, these individuals may be flooded with memories, and those memories may come in the form of intense emotions, clear thoughts, vague images, or unusual physical sensations. Thus, for some parents, the sudden reemergence of their past trauma can be devastating and destabilizing, making them less able to address the needs of their children. Stover and Berkowitz (2005) state emphatically that "it is difficult, but essential, to ascertain the relationship between the parental and child symptoms. The potential for transmission of anxiety symptoms from caretakers to their young children makes it especially necessary for the evaluator not to rely solely on caretaker reports and perform comprehensive assessment of the individual child" (p. 708). I will add that comprehensive assessments of parents are necessary as well since we rely on them so much for information on their child's functioning and improvement.

Parents with newly recovered memories of abuse are thus beginning a parallel process with their abused children. Yet children desperately need a stable, supportive, calm, and confident parent to guide them through their traumatic experiences. Parents may be motivated to help, but they may also feel somewhat incapacitated and may struggle to maintain emotional equilibrium. Thus, it is imperative to provide supportive guidance to parents and encourage them to participate in a structured (sometimes brief) psychotherapy process designed to provide a grounding effect and enable parents to function in the best interest of their children while attending to their own emotional needs. Lieberman and van Horn (2004a) note that there is empirical evidence that symptoms of preschoolers exposed to traumatic situations are predicted by their mother's psychological functioning. They postulate that "it follows that enhancing mothers' ability to help their children cope with trauma should have a beneficial effect on the child's recovery" (p. 123).

CREATING AN ORGANIZED NARRATIVE
IN A RELATIONAL CONTEXT

Professionals have reached consensus about the factors considered relevant and beneficial when working with traumatized children (Lanktree & Briere, 2017; Ford & Courtois, 2013). Among these factors are the following: engaging attachment figures in helping traumatized children; addressing symptomatic behaviors; helping children process traumatic experiences in an effort to restore pretrauma functioning; creating an organized narrative with appropriate cognitive understanding; and encouraging some type of expression. In my experience, expression in young children cannot be limited to verbalizations. In fact, research suggests that expressive therapies may be uniquely suited to retrieving difficult traumatic memories (Nader & Pynoos, 1991; Badenoch, 2008; Chapman, 2014b).

Probably the greatest area of agreement among trauma specialists (supported by research in this field) is that clinicians need to work with traumatic memories head on. Central to that process is helping clients create an organized, sequential narrative of what happened to them. The critical factor seems to be cognitive restructuring that challenges whatever errors in thinking young children might have formed during the trauma (Cohen & Mannarino, 2008; Cohen, Mannarino, & Deblinger, 2006). Having worked with adult trauma survivors a great deal in my early career, it was apparent to me that adults had often grown up with specific cognitive distortions about the abuse, most notably their role in causing or allowing the abuse to continue. Appropriate therapy for complex trauma survivors includes revisiting and challenging thoughts and feelings now firmly in place, formed by young minds with limited perceptual and cognitive abilities. Left untreated, these traumatic experiences had the potential to influence the individual's internal working model. Hence, individuals who have not resolved their childhood traumas, either on their own or through therapy, often have relational difficulties as well as issues with behavioral or emotional regulation, self-esteem, and dissociation, to name a few.

One of the most visible and credible evidence-based treatment programs for children is TFCBT (Cohen et al., 2006). This model engages parents from the outset and provides psychoeducation to both children and families in treatment. The role of parents is fundamental to the successful implementation of TFCBT, a factor that applies to all treatment of child trauma.

I value the inclusion of parents in the process of children's treatment, but with three caveats. First, children should initially have their own individual therapy process using child-centered play therapy; second, parents with histories of abuse need to obtain their own individual parallel treatment prior to participating in conjoint sessions; and third, posttraumatic play must be prioritized and facilitated. Once individual work with both children and their parents or caretakers is completed, a necessary conjoint process is extremely useful to family health. Finally, the timing and delivery of psychoeducation should be carefully chosen; it is best when it includes experiential opportunities.

CONJOINT NARRATIVE SHARING

My particular approach to working with children and their families has evolved over years and was heavily influenced by a systemic understanding of the necessity of family recovery through acknowledgment, processing, and closure. I have seen families err in both directions: a desire to avoid the pain and difficulty of childhood trauma by wanting premature closure, and a complete avoidance of closure. The last-named approach makes the trauma central and explanatory of everything that occurs in the child's development from that point on. Obviously, neither extreme is healthy, and the best way to prevent polarized responses is to work with family systems toward resolution and conclusive actions.

In the conjoint process that seems most relevant, parents and children are prepared to present their perception of events, in whatever way they wish, to each other or other family members. The timing of the conjoint sessions is carefully selected so that participants feel ready to be open and expressive with each other. Questions or worries are identified as well as specific needs for clarification or support. This process is described in depth in Chapter 14 and is highly desirable and conducive to achieving a full family reparation.

THE LARGER FAMILY SYSTEM

Most cases of interpersonal childhood trauma have repercussions beyond the immediate victims. The trauma has ripple effects on the larger family system: grandparents, uncles and aunts, cousins, on both sides of the family. In cases of intrafamilial traumas such as physical and sexual abuse or neglect, there are obvious problem areas that include the child's credibility, how family members feel about keeping family secrets, and familial reactions to contacting legal professionals. Questions arise about privacy, about who should know or be told, about what should be said, and about what resources to tap for help. For cultural reasons, sometimes parents or caretakers have disparate feelings about others knowing and about seeking help. Family members may distrust or feel frightened about involving public service personnel in their lives. Cultural beliefs will influence how family members respond to crisis intervention, their receptivity to formal therapy programs and to other helping services that seem standard responses to CPS concerns. For example, home-based services have grown in popularity and currently get deployed in many cases of childhood trauma. The development of these services was in direct response to concern about removing children from their homes in cases where a parent was willing to respond appropriately to the child. However, for many parents, including home-based services represents an "invasion" of people into their home and often challenges cultural traditions about self-efficacy and family privacy. The reality is that complex trauma elicits many complicated and challenging issues for family members who may feel confused, devastated, ashamed, and ambivalent about designated services and service providers. I usually advocate for carefully assessing which services and service providers appear helpful to the families we are trying to help.

The management of these issues becomes relevant when delivering clinical services to children and their families. Those therapists in private practice will need to become acquainted with the wide array of services that can be activated when children are in the child welfare system. Clearly, when social service or police assessments determine that children are not immediately safe in their homes, they may be moved to foster care or placed with relatives. These removals can cause a great deal of stress. Some children are exposed to families of different socioeconomic resources or to families whose racial make-up or primary language is different from their own. Because children of color make up the disproportionate share of children in foster care, clinicians must keep all these issues in mind (Gil & Pfeifer, 2016).

PROVISION OF PSYCHOEDUCATION

Offering psychoeducation is necessary and desirable, but as mentioned earlier, its timing and delivery strategies must be carefully tailored to the recipients. Individuals have diverse learning styles. Some parents like to read, others prefer to watch videos, and yet others learn by doing. Colleagues often ask me how they can get parents to "buy into" play therapy. My response is that I give the parents themselves an opportunity to do play therapy. Once they have an experience with sand therapy, play genograms, or other brief interventions, they understand the power of play on a very personal level.

An array of psychoeducation can be offered, and many programs focus on providing trauma-specific materials such as "common responses" or "how to promote self-esteem." A videotape produced by the Center for the Developing Child at Harvard University called "Building Adult Capabilities to Improve Child Outcomes: A Theory of Change" (*http://developingchild.harvard.edu/resources/building-adult-capabilities-to-improve-child-outcomes-a-theory-of-change*) promotes systemic work with high-risk children and families. The tape cites a number of different parental capabilities that may need attention, including executive functioning and family regulation. Also discussed are the deficits in our current traditional form of providing psychoeducation: "We are giving information and advice to people who we need to do active skill building with, skill building by coaching, by training, by practice, and we're not doing that." I urge clinicians to search out creative, engaging, and energetic ways, as promoted in this video, to deliver important information and optimize the chances of its integration and usefulness.

It is also important to remember that anxiety interferes with everyone's ability to attend to, and retain, information. Clearly, then, efforts to decrease parental anxiety is critical. Offering too much too soon may be counterproductive. In any case, whatever information clinicians provide must be repeated over and over in different ways. Our integrated approach provides ample options for parents to understand, to reduce anxiety, and to enhance emotional experiences while developing trust in the clinical relationship. Examples of expressive activities are scattered throughout the present book and include sand and art therapy, play, and active dyadic experiences.

ATTACHMENT-BASED WORK

Parents and children will benefit from attachment-based work to establish, strengthen, or reestablish their significant relationship. The term *attachment-based therapy* can include differing approaches. I highly value Theraplay, filial therapy, and Circle of Security (Powell, Cooper, Hoffman, & Marvin, 2013), as well as general family play therapy (Schaefer & Carey, 1994; Gil, 2015c). Each clinician can select from a range of therapies, each of which has specific benefits. Clinicians are encouraged to obtain ongoing training in these important treatments. It's clear that children will have better treatment outcomes when their parents or caretakers feel competent to provide consistent, empathic, trauma-informed care.

REUNIFICATION SERVICES

Clinicians who specialize in working with traumatized children will have opportunities to provide different types of reunification services. Sometimes children who have been in foster care are returned home, and their return is gradual and structured so that visits move from supervised to unsupervised, from public to more private visits, and from brief periods to overnights, to weekends and more. Clinicians may facilitate this process by providing guidance to social services about both parental and child readiness and suggesting supportive services when needed.

If children have been abused or neglected, it is possible that they have had long separations from their biological parents who abused them. It's important to help children achieve personal closure on past events and to assist separated parents and children in determining the optimal type and level of contact. Clinicians must assess what is in the best interests of children and prioritize safety concerns. Relationships with siblings and extended family members may have also been interrupted. Our agency has recently formalized a new service that provides a blueprint for providing reunification services, a topic that has been articulated elsewhere (Gil, 2015a).

We encourage clinicians to consider requests that they provide supervision in parent–child visits. This is a fundamentally different role and function than therapy. This type of monitoring can be provided by paraprofessionals or therapists-in-training who have been trained in the art of observation. Many agencies are currently providing this public service for a fee.

CONCLUSION

Maintaining a systemic approach adds value and necessary substance to the treatment of traumatized children. In addition to offering children a chance to have trauma-focused individual therapy, I believe that family therapy is pivotal to sustaining long-term gains. Family therapy should be engaging, paced, and integrative to maximize positive treatment outcomes. Clinicians are encouraged to seek and identify whatever family-based, evidence-based, and trauma-informed approaches they consider useful to facilitate the family's clinical growth. Several examples of family work are included throughout the chapters that follow.

— *Part II* —
CLINICAL ILLUSTRATIONS

6

The Car Crash

Hillary G. had great enthusiasm as she got into the back seat of her car, hopped onto her booster chair, and strapped on her seat belt. This was her first trip to Disneyland even though she had lived in nearby San Diego for the past 2 years. All her second-grade friends had already visited Disneyland, and each had provided a suggestion for a fun ride. At 7, Hillary was certain this would be her best birthday ever, and although her father could not be with her, Hillary was used to going places with her mother and grandmother.

About 1 hour into their trip, the unthinkable occurred: Mother was hit from behind, lost control of her car, and found herself wheels up, strapped to her seat, with a deployed air bag, and in a great deal of pain. Mother spoke quickly as she described this accident to me, as if she wanted to get all the information out and get it over with. She told me about blood from her head clouding her vision. She also said that her mouth became full of blood, and she felt nauseous and weak. For a while she was disoriented and felt the sting of the air bag on her face. Her pelvis was broken, her leg was broken, and her shoulder fractured as well. She felt overcome and yet struggled to check on Hillary, who was making very faint sounds as she called out to her mother. Within minutes Hillary was in full screams, calling out for her mother in terror. When mother managed to quiet her down, Hillary asked if they were going to die. Hillary cried for her mother to get up and come and get her. Hillary was desperate for touch, and yet she couldn't reach her mother and felt confused by the fact that they were upside down. Mother began to focus on trying to reassure her child in some way, setting aside her own acute panic. She also encouraged her child to pray with her.

INTAKE SESSION

Mrs. G. was an attractive woman in her late 30s who still had the Southern drawl of her native West Virginia. She was cooperative but also struggling with the memory of the event. As she described what happened, her thinking became disorganized, she twitched and moved from side to side, she got teary, she looked away and took long pauses, and she stated that she was unable to provide a lot of details but could send me a letter she had sent to her sister after the accident. I told her that she had given me enough information and asked her to tell me a little about her daughter before and after the accident. I told her I was specifically interested in what she thought was going well and what she thought wasn't yet back to normal.

She didn't describe her daughter too much prior to the accident. When describing Hillary, she said, "She's a great kid, really happy and smart. The accident has changed her. She seems very reticent about everything, she won't take simple risks, like going over and talking to kids at the park. Before the accident, she was much more social, more calm somehow. Now she still wants to sleep in our bed, she has nightmares, and she wants to spend time in her room." Mother said, "This might be funny for you to hear, but I lose her sometimes, and find her cowering in her closet floor, or rolled in a ball under her bed." "It's been 8 months since the accident, and I think she should be over it by now but she still seems to focus on it. Sometimes, she won't get into the car when we're taking her to school."

I asked about Hillary's eating and sleeping patterns and if she was seeing her friends and doing okay at school. Mrs. G. repeated that Hillary was having occasional nightmares and wanted to sleep in her bed. I asked Mrs. G. if she had tried to move Hillary to her own bed, and she said she had not. In part, Mrs. G. offered, she felt more comfortable having Hillary close in case she woke up and needed comforting. Mrs. G. also said that Hillary was often unwilling to get up to go to school, and thus she had fallen behind in her homework. The teachers had noticed Hillary's general anxiety and reported that she seemed very nervous. Hillary's teacher also observed that she often stayed behind, preferring to pass on recess, asking instead, to help the teacher. Given her recent trauma, Hillary seemed to be doing pretty well. Mrs. G. had hesitated to follow the teacher's initial recommendation to take Hillary to therapy but later came to agree that she needed to do so to make sure her daughter was doing okay. When I asked her how her husband had reacted to the accident and how he felt about how Hillary was doing, she remarked that her husband was not psychologically minded. I inquired further, and she said that she and her husband were "not in a good place" and had been talking about a legal separation. "In fact," Mrs. G. said, "he hasn't been around much and didn't show up at the hospital to see me until about 10 days after." Mrs. G. said that Hillary was not hospitalized because "miraculously, she had only minor scratches and bruises," and so she was sent to stay with her grandmother, who lived nearby. Mrs. G. then stated that she herself had sustained a skull fracture, concussion, two broken ribs, a broken shoulder, and a broken ankle, a fact she did not share in our early meetings, perhaps demonstrating her tendency to minimize the impact of the accident. She quipped: "I didn't care that he didn't show right away, and frankly, when he did show, he came in for about 20 minutes and then left on another business trip." Mrs. G. said that Mr. G. and Hillary were not very close and that Hillary spent very little time with him. Toward the end of our session, she confided that Hillary was not Mr. G.'s biological daughter, although Hillary assumed that he was. She stated emphatically that he would not be involved in treatment but had signed authorization forms without asking why they were needed. During the course of treatment, Mr. G. did not return any of my phone calls and expressed no interest in hearing about Hillary or participating in her treatment.

I talked to Mrs. G. about what to say to Hillary about coming to see me, and we scheduled an after-school appointment. I did tell mother that I would have them both come into the first session, so that mother could repeat to Hillary why she was coming to therapy at this time.

I provided typical information to Mrs. G. about what she could expect as I worked with her daughter in therapy. I commented on how resilient her daughter seemed to be, and I explained a little about trauma and how important it is to give children an opportunity to restore order for themselves. I also told Mrs. G. that it would be important for her to have her own therapy because the accident had produced such extensive physical trauma for her as well as psychological effects—driving a car after a car accident creates daily remembrance of what has occurred. When I inquired specifically about how she was doing driving, she responded that she often avoided being in a car, asked her mother to drive her around, opted to walk to work, and had a good friend pick up and drop off Hillary at school. Mother was willing to see a therapist each week during the time that Hillary was in therapy, and I collaborated with Mrs. G.'s therapist over the course of treatment. I also informed her that at some point in my work with Hillary, I would ask her and her husband to join us for conjoint sessions. I was glad that Mrs. G. followed my recommendation for her own therapy since she had a lot on her plate and I did not believe she was addressing her own posttraumatic stress symptoms well enough. She seemed mostly focused on her daughter and hinted that she felt responsible for the car accident and for not being "strong enough" to be responsive to her daughter. In this regard, Lieberman and van Horn (2004a) state:

> When the trauma was the result of an accident, guilt and self-recrimination can have the paradoxical effect of creating parental self-absorption and diminishing attunement to the child's needs. Defensive processes may involve denial, isolation of affect, overidentification with the child, or other mechanisms that interfere with the mother's availability. (p. 117)

My concern with Mrs. G. was her overfunctioning and minimizing the impact of the accident on herself.

BEGINNING THERAPY: FIRST SESSION

Hillary seemed younger than her years, partly because she was so petite. She held her mother's arm and seemed to wrap herself around her. She sat very close to her mother when she came into the office. I introduced myself and then asked her mom to say a little about why she was bringing Hillary to therapy. This was a fascinating process to watch because as much as Mrs. G. had seemed comfortable with talking to her daughter, she hesitated greatly when they spoke together. It became immediately evident that Mrs. G. couldn't quite find the words, and she almost seemed to choke when she talked about the accident in front of her child. Mother looked at me as if pleading for me to help her and I did. I said in a matter-of-fact way that Mrs. G. had told me about the car accident and how the car turned upside down and she couldn't reach Hillary in the back seat. Hillary blurted out, "She was leaking," and I said that mother had told me that there was a lot of blood leaking from her head. "Whew," I said. "Seeing all that blood must have been pretty scary!" "Not for me," she said with a loud voice. I expressed surprise: "Really? What was it like for you?" Hillary then told me that she was "very brave" and that she stayed awake while her mother slept. I then told her that both she and her mom had been through a big crash and it was helpful for her (and Mom) to talk or show how they felt and thought about the crash. Hillary then looked at me with sharp eyes and said, "Are you going to help my mom too?" I reassured Hillary that both of them would get some help for a little while. It was clear that Hillary was taking her cues from Mrs. G., who seemed to feel overwhelmed by memories of the accident. I thought that Hillary's focus on her mother was a plea to help her mother so that mother could help her.

I reviewed with Hillary what Mrs. G. had shared with me about her worries and did so in front of her mother who had asked me to take the lead on this. As I talked to Hillary about her mother's worries, Hillary looked at her mother with concern of her own. I talked to Hillary in developmentally appropriate language, telling her that her mom worried that Hillary was feeling shy, afraid, having nightmares, not wanting to play with her friends, and a little jumpy. "Your mom also told me that sometimes she's looking for you but can't find you and when she does, you're under the bed or in the closet."

It seemed clear that Hillary (and her mother) seemed to be experiencing classic signs of posttraumatic stress, and given that 8 months had passed, mother and teachers were concerned that Hillary had not made adequate progress or stabilized sufficiently from the traumatic event. Mrs. G. was doing better, although she also confided to me that she was glad that "Hillary doesn't want to talk about it all the time. Sometimes, I get so nauseous that I have to go throw up!"

I told Hillary that the first order of business was for us to get to know each other. "Later on," I told her, "I will ask you to show or tell me some more about the accident and how you're feeling now. As a matter of fact, you can talk or show me anything related to the accident anytime you want." I then showed her around the play therapy office. Hillary remained guarded throughout, although she appeared curious as well. I told her that she could decide what she wanted to do and how to spend the time we had together. Mother stayed in the room the full time, which seemed appropriate as she tried to encourage Hillary to look around the room and play with something. I told Hillary that I would look forward to seeing her again and that we would meet on Wednesdays after school. She asked who would bring her to the office, and her mother quickly said that grandmother would be bringing her since she herself had a busy and unpredictable work schedule and it would be hard for her to take off once a week. Hillary asked if her grandmother knew the address and had directions to get here. She was reassured that grandmother would find the office.

SECOND SESSION

The second session went quite differently. Hillary told her grand-mother where to sit and wait for her and told her where she could find some books to read. Her grandmother was a very pleasant, soft-spoken woman who brought her own book to read and seemed happy to wait as long as needed.

Hillary was shy and curious. She talked about her mother being back at work and the fact that she was walking to work, which took her mom almost an hour back and forth. "My mom likes walking a lot!!" she said. Hillary asked about touching things in the office before she touched them, and I reassured her frequently that every-thing in the room was for her to explore. She asked me if I bought all the toys, and I said I did. She seemed impressed with that statement. She then settled on the big wooden dollhouse and began to play with the dolls, setting up a family situation. She grabbed a male figure and called him the dad. She asked if I had another dad with glasses on, and I told her I did not. She said that was okay and then found a little girl doll. "This one has a pony tail like me," she said, and she smiled. She then found a truck and put the dad in the back of the truck. "My dad has a bed in his truck!" "Oh," I said, "your dad sleeps in his truck sometimes." "A lot of times," she asserted, "He's a truck driver and sleeps when he gets tired." Mother had not mentioned this to me but suddenly his being away so much made sense. Hillary then drove the toy truck around the room, making a roaring noise when the truck was gliding along and a screeching noise when the car came to a stop. She also parked the truck in small spaces and said that "dad has to sleep now." She would then go back to the house and continue setting up the furniture and talking about the mom and girl getting ready for school and work. She also asked if there was a grandmother doll, and I found two. She picked one with excitement and said, "This one looks like my Oma." She actually took this doll out to the waiting room at the end of the second session to show to her grandmother who smiled and said there was a resemblance. The second session went quickly, and I noted with interest that the child's play had focused a lot on a family in which the father drove around in a truck a lot.

Hillary seemed excited to come to therapy, and her mother seemed glad that her daughter wasn't complaining about coming or feeling afraid. Mrs. G. kept all her therapy appointments as well, although she had to come in midday, during her lunch break. I collaborated with her therapist and had a monthly meeting with Mrs. G. about Hillary's progress.

EXTERNALIZATION AND CONTAINMENT

About 3 months into therapy, Hillary's play began to take a specific form related to the trauma. It seemed to happen accidentally, but in retrospect, she had always expressed interest in a sandbox in the office that had a second shelf on the bottom of the tray. She had used the bottom shelf as one of the highways for the truck that she drove around. At one point, she had laid on the floor on her tummy and stuck her legs into that bottom shelf, resting comfortably. Each time she did this I noticed how relaxed she looked.

The interesting change was that Hillary got into the small space and held the legs of the box with her hands. She then brought her knees up and shook the tray a little. She started to stretch her legs out, open them, and retract them into her chest. It looked awkward, but she set up a routine in which she would perform this behavior (it looked like crunches) 12 times and then stop. She also asked to put a blanket around the box so that she couldn't see out and I couldn't see her. She told me she liked being in that little space, but she also kept checking to make sure I was still nearby. It dawned on me that this was similar to her being in the closet or under her bed. We started talking through the blanket wall, and I mostly listened to the stories that she told.

Her first story was about how butterflies are born. "Did you know," she said excitedly, "that they know how to break out of the cocoon?" I told her I had heard something about that, and I asked her to tell me what she knew about it. Someone had apparently taught her well. "Then," she said in a hush, "the caterpillar gathers up all her strength and busts down the doors to get out and fly!" I expressed interest in how the caterpillar gathers strength and where it comes from and she said that "all living beings are brave when they want to be free." "Wow," I said, "that's really good to know." I took a chance and asked her if she wanted to draw the inside of a cocoon. "No, thanks," she said sweetly, "I'm busy right now." (Just in case I didn't already know that, she asserted it twice, saying, "Very busy.")

We had many sessions with her inside her handmade cocoon and me on the outside. She seemed to use all her senses as she often noted the smell of the room, the sound of the air conditioning, or muffled voices from our neighbors on the other side of the wall.

I had seen Mrs. G. a few times by now to discuss her daughter's treatment progress and to check in about how things were going at home, and I had asked her to join a session or two since Hillary seemed to want to show her mom what was in the room, particularly her little cocoon. Mom agreed to take a day off to bring her to the appointment, and she also stated that she had heard first-hand from Hillary about the little place she had created in the play therapy office.

JOINT SESSION, RELEASE OF ENERGY, AND ACTIVATION OF RESOURCES

Hillary was so excited that she knocked on the door for me to come out. I was surprised by this first-time behavior but quickly understood the urgency of her request. She brought mother in by the hand, and as I greeted Mrs. G. and pulled up one of the small chairs for her to sit, Hillary had rolled out the sand tray, put the long blankets around the tray, and crawled into the small space she loved. She was silent for a long time. Mother and I spoke together for a few minutes about some recent changes in the office. Then Hillary said, "Be quiet out there, I'm trying to concentrate." I apologized to Hillary and said that mom was now sitting beside her and I would sit at the small table behind her. "Mommy," Hillary said with a very low voice. "Yes sweetie," she said. "Are you okay?" "Of course I'm okay. . . . I'm sitting right here." Hillary said, "But I can't see you!" Mrs. G. and I looked at each other, and it seems in that moment that we recognized what was going on.

"I know you can't see me right now, and I can't see you," Mother said, "but I'm right here." "But are you okay, really?" Mrs. G. reassured her again. Silence. "Mom, can you still hear me?" "Yes, Hillary, I'm right here." Silence. "Mom, how come you didn't answer me when I talked to you in the car that day?" Mom said, "You mean when the accident happened?" "Yes," Hillary said, "I was screaming and screaming, and you didn't answer." "I'm so sorry, Hillary; that was not my fault. I couldn't hear you because I passed out." "What does that mean?" "Well," she continued, "that means that you faint and you can't hear or see anything for a long time." "I thought you died." "Oh, Hillary, I'm so sorry you thought that. We were both really lucky that nothing terrible happened to us." I knew that Hillary would respond to that because she had a very spunky side. "Something happened to me, Mommy, I thought you left me by myself." "I know, Honey, I know that was really horrible. I just meant that I didn't die, neither of us died, and now we don't have to worry anymore." Hillary made her hands grab the inside of the blanket and asked her mother if she could see what she was doing. "Yes," Mrs. G. said, "you're putting your hands on the blankets. "Those aren't blankets," she corrected her, "those are the walls." "Sorry,"

Mrs. G. said, and then she asked if she could try to grab her hands. Hillary was up for that, and they played back and forth trying to find and grab each other's hands. Finally, they ended up holding hands with the blanket in between. Mrs. G. said, "I'm so glad that I found your hand and now I can hold it." Spontaneously, she added, "After the accident, I couldn't move my arms or hands to reach back for you. It was really scary!" "That's okay, Mommy," Hillary said, "I could smell that you were there."

After this session, Mrs. G. and I talked about the session, and I commended her for following Hillary's lead. She wanted to know if Hillary and I had played this game with me, and I said, "No, not in the way she played with you; that was clearly why it was important for you to be here. She seems to want you to really understand how much she needed you and how afraid she was to lose you."

Mother came in with Hillary for an additional six sessions at my request. Mother complied because she understood the importance to her child's ongoing progress. During these sessions, Hillary repeated her play: getting the sand tray ready, ensuring the blankets were securely in place, climbing inside, and having camouflaged dialogue with her mother, who seemed to find increasing strength to "stay with" her daughter without becoming dysregulated and teary. Mrs. G's therapist had been very helpful to Mrs. G. in her own recovery and her progress was evident in the strength she exhibited with Hillary.

In one of the sessions, Hillary used her hands, head, knees, and feet to ask her mother to "guess" what part of her body was behind the screen. Mother played along, offering many guesses before the correct one. Hillary laughed and enjoyed this "hide-and-seek" game quite a bit. I was struck with how Hillary had managed to engage her mother in "finding her" in this play. In the accident, Hillary had been quite affected by her mother being unresponsive and being unable to reach for her.

At some point, Hillary began to show body parts, so she stopped reaching through a barrier; she broke through and started reaching for her mom. In one of those playful moments, Hillary said in a loud voice, "Don't ever pass out again mom, don't do that again!" Mother reassured her that she had "no plans" to pass out in the future. At that point, Hillary crawled out and nuzzled into her mother's lap.

Mrs. G. quietly told her how much she loved her and how sad she was that they had gone through such a scary time. Mother also said how glad she was that they had both been able to get better, and she added, "I'm glad about all the doctors and therapists who have helped us. I was feeling pretty scared for a long time. That was a scary thing that happened." Hillary asked if they would ever have an accident again, and Mom replied: "I hope not. Maybe that was our first and last crash."

AGE-APPROPRIATE RESOLUTION AND CLOSURE

I asked Hillary and Mrs. G. to participate in an art activity that would allow them both to remember and talk about the crash from their different points of view. This intervention was a slight adaptation of Chapman's art therapy treatment intervention (CATTI; Chapman, 2014a) in that I asked each of them for her own set of pictures and I drew the pictures myself rather than asking them to draw them directly. The CATTI is designed "to help children remember, express, and integrate acute traumatic episodes" (Chapman, 2014b, p. 19). The CATTI drawings are (1) a scribble drawing, (2) an event drawing, (3) a helper drawing, (4) a "What happened next?" drawing, and (5) a "leaving and coping drawing," followed by (6) a retelling and (7) closure (Chapman, 2014a).

I opted to draw for them because I had asked both to draw at other times in my work with them and both were acutely ambivalent about anything related to art. Mrs. G. had set the anxious tone about making drawings, and Hillary was quite unwilling to draw or paint at this juncture.

After I made the series of recommended drawings, I simply laid them on the ground in two rows with Hillary's on top and her mother's on the bottom. As we reviewed the drawings, I would pause and wonder aloud about different aspects of them such as sights, sounds, and smells they remembered and how they thought or felt about what happened. Mother's choppy memory reflected her being unconscious off and on. Hillary remembered more details but also felt quite afraid when she first began to remember what had happened. We did some breathing and movement exercises throughout, and I gave both of them a play microphone so that they could expand their voices, even when they were most afraid. I took notes so that I would be able to review the traumatic event with all the information they provided, and slowly but surely, the trauma narrative evolved into a comprehensive narrative of what had occurred from both their perspectives. Both of them also seemed to be able to express empathy to each other and gained an understanding of what each had experienced uniquely, even though they experienced the same event.

We started at "the very beginning." Mom described that they had packed up the car with their suitcases, that they had been very excited about going to Disneyland, and that they both got in the car and headed for the freeway. Mrs. G. remembered that the ground was wet and that it had rained most of the night. She talked about the music that was in the CD player and how they were singing along. Then she remembered someone in front of her stopping without any warning and then suddenly her car started skidding. She said she remembered to turn the wheel into the turn and then hit something. She remembers the car rolling on its side. She screamed and everything happened really quickly and everything went dark. Hillary said that there was smoke, and it got really quiet inside the car and she coughed. She said that she was calling for her mom, but she didn't respond. Mother sat Hillary on her lap at this point and said, "I'm so sorry baby, I wish I had been able to stay awake." Hillary said that there was blood on the seat and that her mom's air bag got red as well. Hillary was upside down and hung on to the sides of the seat belt. Hillary then told her mom that some people were calling out to find out if she was okay ("we had lots of helpers!"). Hillary couldn't talk; she just kept crying because she was terrified and overwhelmed. Then Hillary said she didn't remember much after that but did have a memory of hearing the siren of the ambulance as they were taken to the hospital. She kept yelling for her mom and Nurse Nancy told her that mom was with the doctors and that they were calling her dad. Hillary's grandmother got there within an hour, and Hillary remembered that she felt better when her Oma was with her. As Hillary and her mom talked, the mother reassured her daughter. I made little drawings on a piece of paper that chronicled what they were telling me. After they finished telling me their story, I read it back to them with my little stick drawing pictures. Both of them liked having the pictures, and Hillary laughed at some of the pictures I made. I told them the story from beginning to end, and then I asked Hillary to point at the pictures and tell me the story. As she did that, she added little pieces of information—some about her feelings, some about her thoughts and fears. Mrs. G. held her close and always seemed to say the right things. Then Mrs. G. took her turn.

After this phase of the work, we returned to individual therapy sessions for Hillary and she did more generic play. Much later on, she participated in a series of "goodbye drawings," that included butterflies in flight that she was able to admire in spite of mother pointing to imperfections in the composition. Unfortunately, in about 3 months' time, Mrs. G. asked to come in to tell Hillary that she and her husband were going to get divorced and that her father was going to move out of the house. Hillary cried and asked lots of questions. Mrs. G. seemed very clear that they had many problems and that they were not divorcing her; they were divorcing each other, and eventually Hillary would visit her dad when he had a nice place for her to visit. Some of Hillary's subsequent therapy was about the divorce and specifically, about her feelings of sadness at not seeing her father. Conversely, she was very excited to report that Oma had moved in to the spare bedroom and that she loved having her around.

CONCLUSION

Hillary was a smart, sweet, and vulnerable 7-year-old who had a sudden and unexpected traumatic accident with her mother that left her feeling insecure and anxious. Her mother's presence but inability to protect her and respond to her when Hillary needed her created an attachment disruption. Her mother's temporary incapacitation during the crash had threatened Hillary's sense of safety. This traumatic incident rendered both of them helpless and vulnerable, and neither escaped some severe posttraumatic reactions. Hillary had internalized some of her worries, and she demonstrated the critical underlying struggle with her hiding behaviors in the closet and under the bed.

Trusting that Hillary would eventually show what was on her mind and access reparative strength, I initially followed her lead in individual therapy and allowed her to find her own way toward expression and mastery. The first object she chose was a vehicle, a truck that inadvertently signaled her need for her father, who often drove long distances and slept away from the home. The vehicle that she introduced then explored the play therapy office. She found a way to show her sense of isolation and invisibility as well as her need to be heard, seen, and touched by her mother. This posttraumatic play was critical to this child's recovery and could not have been predicted at the outset of treatment if I had opted to provide her with a pre-scribed protocol of my own, a predesigned way of approaching her. Allowing her to explore and discover what she needed to do was the greatest gift I could give her. Left to her own devices, she created a cocoon environment for herself and covered it with blankets, allow-ing her to have a "can't see, can't hear" environment after the crash. In this way, she eventually heard what her mother had to say and created opportunities for her mother to respond to her, touch her, and comfort her, which she desperately needed and wanted—in fact, compensating in some measure for the isolation that she experienced after the accident.

Treatment for Hillary alone was not sufficient. Her mother needed help to provide her with useful responses. Given an integrated therapy approach, it was possible to refer Mrs. G. to parallel, trauma-focused treatment and to assist her in processing her own traumatic responses to the accident. As she improved, she was better able to turn to her daughter and provide her with calm and clear responses. It became critical for them to remember the event in a more orga-nized way, to cope with the stressor by reaching out and finding each other. A guided conjoint process of facing, documenting, and review-ing the event assisted mother and daughter in obtaining closure and a renewed sense of confidence in self and each other.

7

"When Mommy Comes Back"

*W*hen Millie came to my office, holding the hands of her adoptive parents, she looked quite content, skipping and allowing them to raise her up and jump. She was a small child of 5 years with short, thinning brown hair, which covered some small bald spots on her scalp. She had bright red lips, and as I got closer I saw that she had a small irritation on both her upper and lower lip, apparently from wetting her lips with her tongue. She had a few scars on her fingers and the tops of her hands, remnants of what had likely been a severe case of impetigo. As she approached me, I could see similar scarring on her nose, neck, and ears as well as her ankles.

Mr. and Mrs. L. introduced me to Millie, and she threw her arms around my neck and nearly knocked me over. I learned not to bend down to greet her again. She came with me easily, hardly looking back at her parents, but when the session was over, she gleefully returned to them. I noticed that she had a slight preference for her father's attention, something they had mentioned to me during intake.

INTAKE SESSION

Mr. and Mrs. L., in their late 30s, were pleasant, eager to please, and quite enthusiastic and invested in their new adopted daughter. They emphasized that they had wanted to adopt an older child in the

United States instead of doing what most of their friends had done: pursue an international adoption of an infant. Mr. L. asserted that he and his wife had both been adopted and raised in very happy homes. They wanted to carry on their family tradition of giving to others. They quickly added that they hoped to have their own child in the future but wanted to honor their mutual desire to adopt a child first.

They said that they had limited information about Millie prior to age 3. At 3 years of age, she was placed in a foster home where she stayed for 9 months, and then after the foster father died in a car accident and her foster mother felt she was unable to provide for her, she was placed in another foster home. The second foster home had been a more stable experience for Millie and for two older foster children who apparently required a great deal of attention. The adoptive parents noted that Millie demanded very little of them, and she had to learn to tolerate spending time with them. When she first came to their home, she tended to isolate and "fend for herself." Mrs. L. commented that Millie wouldn't ask to eat when she was hungry, but the mother would find hidden food all over her room. "I wouldn't say she was sneaky, but she sure has light feet and quick speed." She went on to say that Millie seemed to want to stay out of sight and out of the way, and they often found her sitting quietly, seemingly "daydreaming" (a condition I later diagnosed as a dissociative disorder). I asked a few questions about the child's eating and sleeping patterns, which revealed apparent anxiety about having enough food, as well as nightmares and "fretful sleeping." Her parents also said that she seemed more receptive to Mr. L and sought him out more, although she also had a warm relationship with Mrs. L.

Millie had just entered kindergarten and separated without a problem. After kindergarten, Millie's babysitter picked her up from school and took her home for after-school care. During that time, Millie ate lunch, took a nap, and watched *Sesame Street*. The parents both had 9 to 5 jobs and arrived jointly at the end of the day, commuting back and forth to their respective administrative jobs. Millie greeted them warmly and usually sat at the dining room table, while her mother or father prepared something to eat. Her parents told me that they were very curious to see what Millie would do in the playroom because she didn't like playing with toys too much. They said she didn't like to color or make puzzles and preferred to watch

TV. They also had difficulty engaging her in free play with dolls or games. They told me that Millie's teachers found her delightful but a little socially shy and reticent to join in group activities.

BEGINNING THERAPY: FIRST SESSION

After nearly knocking me over with an excited hug, Millie grabbed my hand, and I led her into the playroom. She wasn't overly curious; she didn't touch things or ask questions. Mostly, she waited for direction from me. Once I took her around and showed her all the different toys and activities in the room, she was uncertain what to do. I encouraged her to see what she would like to play with, and she moved over to a crib with a doll inside. When she hesitated to touch the doll, I picked the doll up and held her in my arms. "I like this doll," I said. "I've had her for a long, long time." "She's kind of my favorite," I went on, "because she's really soft, she opens and shuts her eyes, and she often goes to sleep in my arms." I also noted that the doll had black hair similar to hers but not too much like my curly, then blondish hair. I hummed a little song and rocked the doll. Then Millie picked up her blanket. "Does this belong to her?" "Yup," I said, "that's her special blanket; she likes it with her when she sleeps." She didn't want to hold the baby, but she spent time tucking the blanket into the crib, noticing that the crib rocked back and forth, and smelling the blanket. She seemed interested in the doll I held but was reticent to ask for her or accept her when I offered the doll to her. At the next session, she went and kneeled next to the crib and folded the blanket, moving the baby and covering her up. She also rocked the crib back and forth. She was very quiet and hesitant during this play, but she stayed with it for quite a long time. Before she left, I told her I wanted to show her some other things and I opened a drawer that had some babydoll clothes, a bathtub, towels, talcum powder, baby shampoo, and a few bottles and diapers. She looked almost shocked, and she was definitely speechless. She took a step back and asked if she could play with these things next time. "Of course," I said, "they are always in this drawer, and you can decide what to play with." From that point on, her play focused on the baby and caretaking.

EXTERNALIZATION AND CONTAINMENT

Millie's typical activities included hugging and rocking the baby in her arms while humming to her. She also fed the baby in her high chair, gave her a bath with warm soap and water, washed her hair and combed it, and changed her diapers and pajamas. She noticed that one of her pajamas had a spot, and she asked if she could take it home so that her mom could clean it. As this seemed really important to her, I allowed her to take it. She brought it back the following week new and smelling sweet. She was very excited to put the babydoll in it. By now, she was calling the doll her "little baby." She told me that her baby's skin would like the pajamas because they had "soff-ner" smell and they were soft. She paid a lot of attention to the baby's skin. One day she told me that I had to buy some "dess-tin" because that would take away the baby's diaper rash. I went to the pharmacy and picked up some Desitin which she was joyous to use on the doll. She also used a washcloth with great tenderness to clean the baby's body during the wash. In addition, she brought in some hand cream ("my mom gave it to me!"). Mrs. L. was a trained masseuse, and she had given Millie several massages, which she apparently liked and often asked her mom to do.

During some of her play with the doll, Millie found the doctor's kit and was fond of listening to the child's chest, took her temperature, and gave her shots. She also gave her some medicine for her tummy aches. At one point, she said her baby might be having her own baby soon. That didn't last very long, but during the three or four sessions that her babydoll was "preggy," she took extra special vitamins, her tummy was rubbed, and she got "norshing" soups to drink. She used one of the towels as an apron and went to the toy kitchen to make her pregnant doll some soup with lots of good vegetables.

Sometimes the doctors were very kind to the babydoll and asked her how she felt and how she was doing. Other times, the doctors were mean and literally threw the baby across the room. Then in the doctor role, she would instruct the nurse to "please stop that baby from crying."

The above-mentioned play led to another, more distressing type of play: Millie became both the nurturing mother and the neglectful one. She went back and forth between nurturing the babydoll and ignoring her. She sometimes drew with colored pens and paper at the desk. While she colored and talked with me, she would stop and say, "Do you hear something?" "I don't," I replied. I wasn't sure what she was referring to until she said, "That baby better stop crying or else!" I simply stated what I saw: "Mom seems angry at the baby for crying." She agreed that the mother was "pissed!" I then asked what "or else" meant. "Something horrible," she responded." I wondered aloud what this mom could do that would be horrible. "The worst thing ever," she said, "pretend she's not alive." "Oh," I responded, "so this mother might ignore her baby and pretend she's not even alive." She nodded her head and whispered, "Yes." Her play fluctuated in this way for at least 3 months, with both maternal responses being brought to the forefront. Sometimes she would go to the "crying baby" and wrap tissue paper around her head. "She can't breathe, she might die." Toward the end of the session I would ask how the baby was doing and whether she was still crying. "No," she would say sometimes, "she's pretending to be asleep, that way she won't get into trouble." Other times she went into the nurturing mother role and picked up her baby lovingly, rocking her and singing to her. When she was loving, she was very loving, and when she was mean, she was relentlessly so! Each time, I wondered out loud how the baby was doing, what she thought or felt. Eventually, she was able to talk about the baby's feelings, and she assigned her a range of emotions with diverse intensity. She would sometimes yell assertively, "She is berry, berry mad! I don't know why she's so mad at her baby, but she is!" Other times she would say, "Mommy is happy to see her baby. I love my baby and want to keep her with me all the time." Sometimes mother and baby were "best friends"; other times they seemed distant and withdrawn. Millie would state: "She doesn't like her, she thinks touching her is gross." Sometimes the baby was happy and healthy and clean; other times the baby was "gross and smelly."

RELEASE OF ENERGY AND ACTIVATION OF RESOURCES

Millie made some strides in our interactions. Initially, she had hugged me too quickly, asked to come to therapy to see me every day, stalled when it was time to leave and often left in tears, and asked a lot about other children who saw me and if I liked her best. She also wanted to know what other children I played with in "her" room when she wasn't there. Within the first 6 months, she became much more appropriately distrusting and cautious, developing the comfort to ask me questions about what I thought or felt. She would take a sweet tone with me and say, "What do you think (or feel) about that?" She also stayed increasingly connected during our interactions, and her dissociative episodes, both at home and in therapy, were less frequent and briefer—she became more expressive. She had learned to take control at times, while other times, she would ask for my directives. The interactions were far more balanced and appropriate to our therapy relationship.

The other change that evolved over time was that she sometimes brought her mother or father into the session to show them with pride some aspect of her play. She was very purposeful in what she shared with them. She never shared negative feelings or painful situations, perhaps not wanting to reveal intense emotions in front of them to protect either herself or them. The parents had remained cooperative and attentive throughout Millie's treatment, and we met once a month to review ongoing challenges as well as improvements in Millie's eating, hoarding food, and sleeping patterns. Overall, it seemed that Millie was improving as she utilized posttraumatic play in an effort to process some of her memories with her mother. Eventually, she asked me if I knew her mother, and she wondered what had happened to her. I thought it was important for Millie to know something about her mother's disappearance. I realized at this moment that I had not tracked information about Millie's birth parents. I became aware that I knew more about her prior two foster parents than I did about Millie's mother. When I asked Mr. and Mrs. L., they noted that Millie's mother had been young and drug addicted and had neglected Millie. They reminded me about her neglect, Millie's nonorganic failure to thrive, and her multiple caretakers. They noted her small weight, her physical scarring, the fact that there were old and healing injuries in her body. She also had many other physical ailments resulting from malnutrition that were addressed as soon as she was placed in a stable foster home. I asked Millie's adoptive mother if she would give me permission to check with the adoption agency for any other information about the birth mother. From my first phone call I learned that her mother had died from a drug overdose shortly after Millie was placed in foster care and that her birth father was listed as "unknown." The social worker insisted that Mr. and Mrs. L. knew about mother's death and told me she would be in touch with them.

I talked to the parents about what I had learned; they had already talked to the adoption worker who had reminded them that they had already told her about Millie's birth mother dying. Mr. and Mrs. L. were quite taken aback when I suggested that this was important information for Millie to know. It has been my experience that children who are adopted need the truth and an opportunity to achieve some kind of closure about their birth parents. Otherwise, it seemed possible to me that Millie might continue to wonder about her mother and feel unsettled about whether she was permanently in the care of Mr. and Mrs. L. It seemed particularly relevant to inform Millie of her mother's death since she was working hard to deal with her past relationship to her birth mother, remembering, playing out, exposing herself to her needs, and nurturing herself. It had become clear that as Millie played out her mother's inconsistent care, her frightening and fleeting nurturing behaviors, and her extreme neglect, she was also letting go of past memories as she was beginning to accept the caretaking that was now consistently available to her. A new treatment goal was to facilitate Millie's connection with Mrs. L. specifically on the topic of mother–child relationships, which had now become intertwined in Millie's mind. I secretly hoped that the next time Millie brought her mother or father into her session she would feel a little less defended (or protective of her parents).

As soon as I saw Millie's willingness to begin to show more of herself to Mrs. L. (Millie appeared less inhibited), I talked to Mr. and Mrs. L. about adding conjoint sessions in a second meeting each week. The mother agreed easily, and the father said he would be interested as well. Since the father's attachment to Millie seemed more secure and less anxious, I asked that he participate after Mrs. L. had a chance to have some mother–daughter sessions.

Millie was excited to hear that she would be coming to see me twice, once by herself and once with her parents. Apparently, she had asked many times about her own session and wanted reassurance that it would continue without interruption. Prior to starting the conjoint sessions, she asked me, "What are we going to do with my mom?" I told her that she could decide how to spend time with her mom. When Millie asked me why her mother would be coming into therapy with her, I told her: "You play a lot about mommies and babies. I think it might be a good idea for you and your mom to play together about mommies and babies." I could see the wheels spinning in Millie's head, but she didn't ask anything more. Instead, she returned to her play and took inventory, reminding me that I had offered to buy some new diapers for the dolly. I told her I would do that before her mother came in with her.

JOINT SESSIONS:
AGE-APPROPRIATE RESOLUTION AND CLOSURE

Millie was subdued during the first joint session and wanted to show her mother around, holding her hand, showing her all the toys she had played with, where she drew, and telling her some idiosyncratic facts about the room: the air conditioning makes a big noise when it goes on; sometimes you can hear people walking outside, but we have a noisemaker we can turn on. Mrs. L. was very attentive to her daughter, seemed excited to look around, asked questions, and was supportive and sweet. Millie showed her mother all kinds of things but kept her babydoll tucked under a blanket. The next few sessions she followed suit, until finally, in the middle of one of the sessions, Millie told her mother that they were going to give someone a bath. "Someone?" asked her mother. "Shhhh," she said, looking over to me, "Don't tell her." She prepared the bath, set out the towel, shampoo, soap, and new babydoll clothes. She proudly introduced her mom to the doll: "Here she is, Mom, *she's* getting a bath today." Mother shook the little doll's hand and then asked if the water wasn't too cold. Millie agreed and got a little more warm water.

And so it went. This sequence of play included mother fully. At first, Millie asked for her mother's help and told her what to do. In subsequent sessions, she simply showed her mother how she played with "her baby," and the sessions were reminiscent of her earlier play. Her mother had asked me how to respond, and I simply told her to stay attentive and follow Millie's directives. Mrs. L., who had seemed a little distant when I first met her, could not have done a better job of being emotionally connected to her child and witnessing her daughter's experience without judgment.

A typical session went like this: Millie took out the babydoll and placed her in the high chair. "Mom, get the baby some lunch please, I'll put her in her chair." Mrs. L. went to the food bin and prepared some food on a plate while Millie put the bib on the baby. "She still likes her bottle, and she likes to eat lunch food too!" She would ask her mother to feed the baby. Mrs. L. fed the baby and made Millie laugh by making airplane noises and landing food in the doll's mouth. Millie stood next to Mrs. L. as they fed the baby. "Mom, wait," she would say, "blow the food . . . it's too hot!" Mrs. L. would oblige quickly, telling Millie that she was such a good mommy and took care of her baby very well. At first, I wasn't sure how Millie would respond to her mother's interpretation of her as the mother and the baby as hers. But Millie did not correct her mother. Two weeks after this session, Millie said, "Your grandma is going to feed you today." Mrs. L. said, "Grandma loves her baby and her baby's baby."

On another occasion Millie asked her mother if she had a good mommy when she was little. Mrs. L. said: "Oh, yes, she was a wonderful mommy. She adopted me when I was just a baby." "Were you drinking a baby bottle?" Millie asked and mother said, "Yes, I was only a few days old when my mom adopted me." "What happened to your other mommy?" "I really don't know, Millie; no one ever told me anything about her." I sat surprised, realizing that this was the missing puzzle piece about why Mrs. L. had forgotten the information about the death of Millie's mother. Millie seemed really quiet and apparently asked Mrs. L. more about her mother when they got home. "Do you miss your other mommy?" Mrs. L. told me that she didn't know how to respond but remembered my advice to tell the truth. Mrs. L. told Millie that she never missed her because she never knew her. Then Millie said that she knew her other mommy when she was little. Mrs. L. asked if Millie remembered much about her other mommy, and she said "No," after which Mrs. L. dropped the comment. Later that night, Mrs. L. left me a voice mail saying that she agreed it would be helpful to let Millie know that her mom was dead, but she didn't know how to do it. We had a family session to review the couple's beliefs about death and how they would like to describe this to their daughter. They agreed to tell her that when people die, their hearts stop beating and the body dies but that each person has a soul that then leaves the body and goes to heaven. They seemed comfortable about having this conversation with Millie and did so easily. Mrs. L. called to say all had gone well and that Millie seemed to understand but hadn't asked any questions. They were unclear what feelings she had, if any.

At our next session, Millie was quiet and went through her usual routine with the babydoll, this time lingering for a long hug. She kept fussing with the baby's hair, and I asked how the baby was feeling. She told me the baby was sad because her mother had gone to heaven. I reassured the baby that it was okay to be sad and that even though her mom was in heaven, there would be another mommy on earth that would take care of her. Millie looked down for a while and then asked if my mom was dead. I told her she was not. Then Millie asked if Mrs. L. would die. I responded that everyone dies sometime but usually people live for a long, long time and they die when they've lived a long life. "Remember, your mom is your baby's grandma." "Yeah," she responded. "Well, your mom will probably live long enough to maybe have other grandbabies someday." I realized this was an abstract thought, and to this day I don't know if Millie understood what I was saying. She didn't ask more and I didn't volunteer more. I did let Mr. and Mrs. L. know what she had asked, and Mrs. L. found different ways to reassure Millie and focus on all of them growing older, having more holidays together, and going on vacation the following year.

Millie's play in both the individual and joint sessions continued for a few months. Eventually, the doll play became less present and took less time. This was replaced by her interest in other things such as using the sandbox, painting pictures, playing games with me, and making arts and crafts. Slowly but surely, Millie became more outgoing, more confident, and well attached to both her parents. In addition, her symptoms decreased significantly, so that we began to talk about termination. It was during this time that Millie's processing became deeper and her closure with her mother became clearer.

ENDING THERAPY

Millie had an important experience during termination. After our 2 years together, she and I had become important to each other. I had told her from the outset that I worked with children only for brief periods of time, and then they didn't come to see me anymore. I said

I would let her know when I thought it was becoming time to end our sessions; her initial reaction was to regress. She cried in my lap and told me she didn't want to stop coming to see me. She told me she didn't want to say goodbye and wanted to come until she was 10! This was tough for both of us, and by now, Mrs. L. was also convinced that Millie should keep seeing me throughout elementary school. I discouraged this notion, reminding the parents that they were doing just fine and that Millie was thriving in their care. They overattributed her progress to therapy, and I acknowledged therapy had been a part of what had helped her but that much more had come from deep inside Millie.

I told Millie that for now, we would meet every other week, and the week we did not see each other, she and her parents could spend the therapy time doing something special together. I had taught her parents some Theraplay techniques, and they found the dyadic experiences fun and energizing. Millie seemed somewhat consoled knowing that she would do something special with her parents. Then she asked me what I would do. I told her that I would think of them having a good time.

We did bimonthly sessions for about 3 months, then moved to monthly appointments, and next to quarterly ones. Each time we made a change, Millie expressed sadness, and I told her how well she was showing exactly what she felt inside. I reminded her that when I first met her, she didn't like to talk about her feelings and that sometimes she pretended she wasn't having any.

When we moved to monthly meetings, I sent Millie a little card in between sessions. Mr. and Mrs. L. told me how excited she was to receive mail addressed directly to her, and she insisted on making me a thank you picture which she delivered at our next meeting.

Millie and I started working on a termination book. We chronicled what was going on when I first met her, how she was doing now, and what she was looking forward to in the future. She transported the book back and forth until our last meeting. By then, we had talked about how we were keeping each other in our hearts and minds while we were apart, and she often told me of times she had thought of me.

We had a celebration session with her parents to say goodbye. We planned it carefully and had her favorite dessert and balloons. She wrote me a sweet note, and I gave her a little present. She opened it and gave a big smile when she saw it. "Thank you, Dr. Gil, I will keep it always." She showed it to her mom and then said, "I don't want to take it out of the box, I want it to stay new forever!" The little present was a small doll in a high chair with miniature food. A year after we had our last session, her mom told me the box remained unopened. She also shared the news that she would be having another baby in a few months and that Millie couldn't wait to become a big sister!

CONCLUSION

Millie had experienced severe neglect from her birth mother, which she was able to play out by using babydolls in our play therapy office. She seemed to need to externalize the difficult and hurtful experiences that she remembered and had kept buried deep inside her. At the same time, externalizing the difficult experiences gave way to her accessing internal resources, and she herself provided nurturing care to the doll, conjuring up positive dyadic images of appropriate parent–child care. I believe that Millie was using posttraumatic play in order to organize her experiences of a parent who had neglected and eventually abandoned her, as well as a new adoptive parent, who seemed willing and able to provide appropriate care. One way to understand this was Millie's desire to clarify events in her own mind so that she could gain closure and be able to welcome her current parent figure. Millie herself guided the process throughout her therapy, and I provided a safe and predictable environment for her. I also invited her parents to attend conjoint sessions so that they could witness some of her play and could support her more fully. In addition, I coached the parents in how to tell Millie about her birth mother's death, so that Millie could undergo appropriate grieving and worry less about her mother returning to take her away from her current home. Millie's play and her parents' involvement and guidance allowed this young child to face traumatic memories in her own way, to organize and clarify sequential experiences, and to achieve closure on her early childhood experiences. Working in this way allowed her to be more receptive to parental nurturing and caretaking from her adoptive parents.

8

"Daddy Hits Me When I'm Really Bad"

*D*ot was a sweet little 9-year-old who had been in foster care for the past 4 years. She had a collateral plan of reunification and adoption, and it was unclear if either biological parent would make the necessary effort to meet the demands of the court sufficiently to have their child returned to them. The DFS had done everything it could to engage the parents in mental health treatment, addiction services, anger management classes, and couple therapy. The mother had been intermittently receptive, whereas the father had been flat-out resistant. The parental relationship had been volatile and interrupted by many separations, multiple partners, and brief and intense reunions. Dot had been through the ringer: She was known to the DFS since she was very young and had been in foster care twice before. The mother always seemed to rally after she became frightened that she would lose her children. Dot's siblings were also in foster care— the eldest in residential care and the other two together. The siblings had periodic contact; parent–child visitation also occurred when the mother was able to get transportation and prioritized her children. The social worker had confided that she remained convinced that the DFS would be filing for termination of parental rights, particularly because the foster family had expressed interest in adopting the set of siblings, even while recognizing that these children would have special needs.

The DFS's paper trail was dense with reports of physical abuse, domestic violence, and drug and alcohol abuse. Dot, in particular, was singled out for chronic and relentless physical abuse by her father. When I met Dot, many of her injuries were immediately visible, with lots of marks on her arms, hands, and thighs. Given that the intake concern was self-harm, I was not surprised to see that Dot had an array of old, healing injuries as well as fresh, new injuries, some of which looked inflamed or infected.

INTAKE INFORMATION

I met with Mrs. W., the DFS's social worker assigned to this case. Her passion and concern were welcome and immediately evident in the way she described how each of the children was doing in foster care. She noted that Dot's 14-year-old brother had been sexually victimized by some men who stayed in the home. He had developed sexually aggressive behaviors and was currently in residential care for teens with offending behaviors. Dot's other two siblings were a boy of 6 and a girl of 4. These two children had been removed from their mother's care when they were 2 and 4, respectively, and they lived together with a couple who was devoted to them and wanted to adopt them.

Mrs. W. described Dot's chronic history of child maltreatment, one that made me wonder why parental rights had not already been terminated. But then she proceeded to tell me that Dot's mother had also grown up in foster care and was a "lost soul" who barely had a chance to improve her life because she had come "under the spell" of her husband at a very young age, 14 to be exact. She then described the biological father in highly negative terms but also noted that he had been in the juvenile justice system since his early adolescence and had also lived in group homes most of his life. His minor legal problems grew as he matured into a gang member and later into an abusive husband and father with persistent drug issues. Dot's father was combative with the DFS, his probation officer, the arresting officers, and the judge. The oppositional conduct disorder of his youth had escalated to full-blown sociopathic behavior, which had landed him in trouble most of his adult life. Because of this basic disregard for authority figures, he consistently refused help, felt entitled to treat his wife and children as he wished, and demonized the department and its "witch-hunt" of his family. She also stated that he had been arrested trying to force his way into her office and had been relentless with his threats and "general animosity." She said the judge was fed up, and she did not anticipate that this father would be given more chances. Mrs. W. was more empathetic to the mother but also emphasized that she was "a child raising children, incapable of protecting them."

Mrs. W. told me that Dot had been in treatment before, but the therapist had gone on maternity leave and had opted not to return. Dot had been treated for "reactive attachment disorder," which appeared to be a premature diagnosis since she had made a good adjustment to her new foster parents. Mrs. W. was now concerned that Dot was hurting herself, putting rubber bands around her wrists so that they left marks, and had held her hand to a lit candle. The foster parents were unable to attend, but they had filled out the Child Behavior Checklist (CBCL), which provided additional details about Dot's persistent self-injurious and other impulsive behaviors. I had also talked to the foster parents, who seemed quite invested and concerned about their ward.

BEGINNING TREATMENT: FIRST SESSION WITH DOT

Dot was alone in the waiting room when I came out to see if she had arrived. Apparently, her county driver had dropped her off, told her to wait for me (she had verified that I was in the office), and had left. Another driver would be picking her up. Thus, when I came out to see her, she was sitting quietly in a big chair, holding her jacket and a stuffed rabbit. I asked her if she was Dot and I told her who I was. She came with me easily and looked around the play therapy office, quickly asking if I had a "Connect Four" game. I told her I did not. "Miss Linda had one of those. That was our favorite." From this point forward, Miss Linda visited our sessions through Dot's conversation, and it seemed to me there had been a lack of closure in that therapy relationship. Eventually, she confided that she was "mad" at Miss Linda because she promised her she would come back after the baby "came out." She also told me that when Miss Linda came back, she wouldn't see me anymore.

I asked her why she thought she was coming to see me, and she shrugged, "I don't know, I always go to therapy." I told her that this time it was because her foster parents were worried that she was hurting herself and making marks on her body. When I said that, she covered her arms a little but then went on to continue looking around. When I asked if Miss Linda had a sand tray, she said no, "but she was going to get one." This was another consistent behavior in Dot: she protected the memory of Miss Linda fiercely and never wanted her to come out on the short end of anything!

During the first session, Dot spent time exploring the office and checking me out. She asked if I had kids, if I bought all the toys, how many kids I saw in addition to her, and whether I knew Miss Linda (in fact, I did, but I never told her that). I also knew that Linda's child had been born with a congenital heart problem and had numerous surgeries in her first months of life, but I never told her that either.

She asked who would be taking her home, and I said "a driver." She asked which one, and of course I didn't know. The driver was late, and I told her I would wait with her downstairs until he or she arrived. Traffic at our office was quite intense in the afternoon, and drivers were almost always late, which had precipitated us writing a policy requesting that the drivers stay in the building. I communicated that to the driver, and she told me she would not leave the office during the session and, from that point forward, stayed in the waiting room.

The first session was uneventful except for one exchange. Dot seemed interested in the sand; however, she had an open sore slightly above her wrist, and so I told her that just until her sore got better, I would give her some gloves to wear in the sand. She asked what would happen if the sand got into the sore, and I said that it would irritate her sore, which could get infected. She put on the gloves in cooperative fashion, but I noticed that when she took them off she stuck her hands in the sand quickly and sprayed sand on her sore. I quickly took her to the sink and poured water on it. "The sand may irritate your sore. Your sore needs a chance to heal, so it's better not to get sand in it." She didn't respond but allowed me to pour warm water on her arm. As she left, I told her that it was important to let her skin heal and to take care of herself. "Okay, okay" she said, sounding irritated at my comment.

REENACTMENTS

During the next 2 months (eight weekly sessions), I found Dot to be a little irritable, dysregulated, and impulsive. She brought the following behaviors into the room for my immediate response:

1. She often brought in or found rubber bands in my office. She disguised putting them on and twisting them so that they became tight. Obviously, I stayed vigilant to this behavior but noted the sneakiness with which she did this, in plain sight, but hidden. When she removed the rubber bands at my insistence, she took her index finger and rubbed the mark on her wrists.

2. She often dug the sand, so that she filled the area under her fingernails. At home, the foster mother told me that she had found her rubbing the sand into her open sores.

3. She bumped into things in my office, sometimes bruising her thighs. No matter how many times I moved or covered things, she managed to bump into something, much as she reportedly did at her foster home.

4. After she did something that I had told her not to do (usually something dangerous—for example, climbing onto the sandbox when it was covered and jumping off), she appeared frightened about what I would do. Lots of times she would ask if I was mad at her and if I was going to hit her. I reassured her I would not hit her or let her hit me, but she kept asking. When she knowingly misbehaved, she seemed earnestly panicked for a few minutes.

5. She noticed all sharp objects and always plunged them into her skin quickly—so much so that I had to do a quick review of the room before starting our sessions. Because I shared my play therapy office with others, this seemed important to do. Often, others brought things into the office or left things out that could be dangerous. Dot had good investigative skills, and we usually found something that needed to be put away.

6. When she burned her hand at her foster home, she showed me the round shape of the burn and its color. She was clearly enthralled with whatever marks she could create on her skin.

7. Finally, the foster parent reported that Dot was masturbating by sticking things inside herself; the parent had discovered this when Dot injured herself and bled into her underwear. The foster mom took her to a doctor, and Dot described what she had done without inhibition.

TREATMENT INTERVENTIONS

From the outset, this was more of a directive case. It became clear to me from the first session that this child was asking for a lot of limits and was bringing the issues of abuse into the therapy office. Too often, children who are physically abused chronically will have an array of confusing thoughts and feelings. Their relationship to pain appears slightly different. Sometimes pain triggers a dissociative response that can feel helpful to the child (Dot would say, "I'm outta here"). In these cases, children don't look like they are feeling pain, and they may underreport pain or simply have the experience that it is numbed.

Other times, they feel exaggerated pain with minor or absent provocation, respond in an extreme way (crying and yelling), and elicit caretaking responses from others (which they sometimes accept or reject).

The other interesting dynamic at play between Dot and me was that she seemed to be asking for clarity about my responses—what I would do or say, how I would handle her misbehaviors, and whether or not I would repeat abusive patterns. Dot was also testing object permanence: Would I stick with her? Would she have to leave prematurely? How could she remain loyal to her previous therapist while being receptive to me?

Another gripping dynamic was her self-injury, which I interpreted as her attempt to gain mastery. An adolescent I had worked with earlier, who had a history similar to Dot's but who had been sexually abused as well, articulated this dynamic pretty well: "I decide who hurts me, I decide when to start and stop it. I'm in the driver's seat!" This adolescent had learned that there was something useful about reenactments. In her case, it led to her putting herself in harm's way and suffering a number of physical assaults.

So therapy with Dot had at least three concurrent and compelling dynamics: attachment issues, behavioral reenactment of abuse in both behavior and action, and self-injury. This child not only engaged her therapist in setting limits and keeping her safe, but she also hurt herself and developed a fascination with the marks she put on her body. Thus, my work with her required me to be more directive as well as much more focused and patient. In addition, her self-injury was compulsive and potentially dangerous and unhealthy.

This was clearly a case of posttraumatic play that was being acted out in a unique fashion, turned inward, toward herself. Many of the victim–victimizer dynamics were being challenged within the context of the therapeutic relationship. The foster mother reported having seen some of the same behaviors surface within her relationship as well, particularly as our treatment continued and Dot faced other stressful life events.

In the middle phase of therapy, which lasted about 9 months, I used a variety of interventions, many of which are listed below. During this phase of therapy, Dot had to testify in court, and the court ordered that she be freed for adoption. That process took another year to finalize, but her life outside therapy presented numerous challenges. At times, her symptoms decreased or disappeared altogether but then reappeared during stressful times.

Bracelet Intervention

I thought it would be useful to address Dot's injuries at the wrist and her tendency to make this marking using rubber bands. I told her that I had noticed that she did that, and I wanted to see if we could do some other things in addition. I have learned that it is not useful to tell children to stop behaviors because it engages them in a power struggle. I assume that if they were motivated to stop the behavior on their own, they would. Instead, I find it more beneficial to try to add some new behavior and whenever possible to help children show me what their motivation is, or I suggest some ideas about how I understand what they are doing.

In Dot's case, I said something like this: "I understand that it's better for you to be in control of making marks on your skin, rather than having someone else do it." She looked up at me and then looked away. I went on to say that so far she had figured out a way to make marks, but I hoped we could find a way to make marks without causing actual injuries to her skin. I brought out some yarn, had her pick a color, and we made a bunch of bracelets together. We measured her wrist and created some bracelets that were "too tight," "too loose," or just right. I asked her to slip on a bracelet when she had the urge to pinch her skin or make a mark with rubber bands. In addition, in the next session, I pulled out a "too tight," "too loose," and "just right" bracelet, and I told her I wanted to make a face. I presented her with plastic eyeballs, noses, and mouths. The nose and mouth were little stickers, while the eyeballs were stickers of different colors and sizes that I had purchased at a crafts store. We spent that session making three faces on different pieces of paper. She brought out some yarn to make hair as well. When she started to pick the mouths, I asked her to make sure they were open versus closed mouths because I heard that these three were going to be interviewed on a TV show. She went with the flow, neither objecting nor asking more about what I meant.

I then told her that she could be my assistant and take notes. I gave her a clipboard and paper and pencil and asked her to take whatever notes she had or to write down whatever questions she had. She acquiesced and sat down while I set up the faces. I then played a little music from my phone and announced that the show would be interviewing these three bracelets and asking them what it was like to be them.

When I talked to the "too loose" bracelet, I pretended to repeat her answers or ask clarifying questions. The dialogue went something like this:

> "So, what's it like to be a bracelet that is simply 'too loose' on people"?
> "What's that you say? People lose you all the time?"
> "That must be hard on you. . . . What? You *hate* it when that happens?"
> Dot added, "I bet you don't like it when people lose you and they don't come looking for you." I thought this quite profound.
> "Who's your favorite wrist?" I asked, smiling. Then I said, "Little girls, really? I know some little girls."

The next questions were addressed to the "just right" bracelet, and this line of questioning was noneventful. We then moved on to questioning the "too tight" bracelet, and I took the lead.

"So 'too tight' bracelet . . . what's going on? How come you like
    to fit wrists too tightly?"
"How did you get to be too tight?"
And the most productive question: "What would you like to say
    to the wrist? What would you like the wrist to know?"

I waited for a few minutes, stating what a good question this was, and I wondered out loud what the response might be.

Dot became very animated, took the piece of paper with the "too tight" bracelet, and raised her voice holding the paper in front of her face. "You are a bad girl, you don't listen, you drive me crazy. I have to teach you a lesson, I'm sick of telling you to stay put!! Now you'll be sorry!!" She stood with the paper in front of her face. "Wow," I said, "that's one angry bracelet!" She whispered under her breath, "Yeah, but she makes me mad; she's really bad." I asked what the girl did to make the bracelet mad, and she said "everything." I then asked what happened when the "too tight" bracelet stayed on. "Sometimes," Dot said spontaneously, "my dad would tie me to the bed, and I would try to get free and my wrists would get all red." I told her I was really sorry to hear about this. I asked how she took care of her red wrists, and she said she didn't; she would just cover them up so nobody would see them. I then asked how often this happened with her dad, and she said "lots of times." I then asked why she thought he did that and she responded that she was really bad. When I asked what she did that was bad, she again repeated "everything," but she was unable to give an example. I told her that it sounded like she had decided there was only *one* explanation for what happened. "I don't know," I said, "lots of times there are two, three, or even four different explanations about why things happen." "What?" she asked. "I don't know," I said, resisting the temptation to give immediate information. "How about this? Let's put our heads together, and you think of at least one other explanation, and I'll think of another. Next week, we can see what we came up with. I'll write it on a piece of paper so I don't forget."

The following week she brought a folded piece of paper and I had mine. She handed it to me, and I showed mine to her. I told her I would read them out loud, and she sat to listen attentively. Her piece of paper had the following words: "She's bad and cries a lot." Mine said: "I don't know how to be a parent without hitting my children." "Ah, ah," she said, "he was a good daddy, I did bad things." "Like what?" I asked again, and she answered that she didn't know. I told her that lots of kids who are hurt think that they are hit because they are bad. Then I said, "If kids do something they shouldn't do, parents need to teach them, show them what's right; they don't have to hit them. Kids are kids. They need to be taught right from wrong; they're not born knowing that." She listened and turned away. That day her play was very hectic, and she went from thing to thing, almost like she had nervous energy. Her foster mother wrote me midweek to let me know that Dot was unusually defiant for a few days following the session. She asked me if something had happened. My response was, "Sounds like she's just checking in to make sure no matter what she does, you won't hit her."

Clay Intervention

I told Dot that her mom had mentioned her taking sand home and rubbing it into her sores. I told her I noticed that I had less and less sand in my box and that I needed her to keep the sand in the box.

I then told her that her mom and I both wanted to help her keep from picking at her sores because, as she knew, they would get infected, turn redder, and form lots of big scabs. I then invited her to use some clay to make an infected sore. She used red clay and flattened out pieces of black and brown for the scabs, using yellow for what she called the "pus." Once again, I asked her to speak for the infected sores, and this time she got behind a puppet theater and put the clay sore in the front. She spoke loudly this time: "What I got to do to make you notice me?" "I need you to take care of me; I need you to make me better!!" I then asked her to change places with me and when I used her words, she responded. "There, there, you're going to be okay, you're going to get better. I know you're scared but sometimes people stick with you, no matter what." She repeated this over and over again, and then she asked to go see her foster mother who had brought her to the session. When she got out to the waiting room, she climbed on her lap and no words were spoken.

Regarding her "accidents" I would always stop and take notice and make sure I checked her body to see if she was okay. We had a routine in which I always stopped what I was doing, showed interest in where she was hurt, and she would try to move away quickly. I would pull her back gently, telling her it was very important to me to make sure she was safe. I even started moving furniture around to remind her that I was thinking about her and her safety.

Slowly but surely, her testing behaviors decreased, and she seemed to grow more secure in the therapy relationship as well as in her relationship to her foster mother. Thus, when the time came for the termination of parental rights hearing, she wrote a letter to the judge stating that she wanted to be adopted by her foster mother and now understood that her father was wrong to hit her. As for her mother, she wrote, she could not take care of anyone, including herself, and certainly not a baby who needed to be kept safe and protected. The termination hearing proceeded quickly, and the adoption also went off without a hitch.

Termination with this child went slowly and proceeded in a structured way. Because she had so many disruptions in her life and hardly an opportunity for organized goodbyes, I structured a gradual decrease in visits so that she could integrate the concept of leaving with closure.

CONCLUSION

Traumatized children experience stress that overwhelms adaptive coping strategies and often elicits defensive mechanisms that are central to their survival. As they grow older, they may inadvertently bring the trauma to the forefront of their lives through behaviors or play that is reminiscent of aspects of the trauma, especially if they are abused when they are very young. This reenactment or repetition suggests unresolved trauma, but it may be out of their conscious awareness. Posttraumatic play allows them to externalize their worries, and often processing follows.

This chapter has discussed how post-trauma play and post-trauma behavior can be interrelated. This type of behavior often needs outside help to reach a safe resolution and directive approaches and interventions may become necessary.

9

When Posttraumatic Play Doesn't Emerge Naturally

BEGINNING THERAPY

This unusual case involved a 9-year-old girl named Debbie, who was forced into prostitution by her parents. I remember being shocked when I met Debbie, who seemed just like any other girl her age except for her eyes and her demeanor. Her eyes looked incredibly sad and tired, and it was evident upon meeting her that she wasn't comfortable or easy. She got into a chair quickly and wrapped her arms around herself, literally. She wasn't combative at all, and she complied with all my requests. At the same time, she was distant and disengaged, as if she was playing the role she thought I expected her to play. She glanced around the room with a look that appeared to show both feelings of disdain and longing. I sensed that she wanted to touch things but wouldn't let herself do so. (She confirmed this intuition months later when she described herself as "frozen, like a snowman, watching people walk by.")

Her posture and routine was consistent for a couple of months: She held herself in the same easy chair for about 2 months before she began to relax. During those first 2 months I read police and DFS reports, and I talked to her current teachers and foster parents. The police investigator called me to inquire about her health—it appeared that Debbie elicited much concern from those who came into contact with her, and she had a team of four or five professional cheerleaders (teachers, social workers, attorneys, recreational thera-pist), hoping that she would be able to recover from her treacher-ous past. Her teachers and foster parents also reported a compliant child who kept to herself and was very self-sufficient. Debbie was a youngster who could remain off everyone's radar screen because she seemed asymptomatic and was emotionally and behaviorally regu-lated and acquiescent. Even the tutor assigned to her after regular school hours thought she was a "special girl," eager to learn but officially very behind in her academic functioning. The school had found few records, partly because she had been registered by differ-ent names in different jurisdictions and partly because there were periods of time when she had not attended school and stayed home by herself.

Debbie had a journal someone had given her, and she either drew or wrote in it most days, filling it mostly with clear and evocative poetry. Her calligraphy and command of the language were impres-sive. I kept a note she wrote me when she moved away: "You did not look away. You did not raise your hand. Your eyes asked for nothing. Your voice always the same. Thank you."

I was happy to hear she had some method of expression since she seemed to alienate herself from personal relationships. I made a men-tal note that she stayed far from her foster father, perhaps because she was nervous around males, afraid they might become abusive. Her strong wish to go unnoticed made sense when I read the police report and her mother's statement that she brought tricks up to the apart-ment and they could choose her or "the kid." My impression that she wanted to blend into the woodwork made absolute sense to me. Not being seen guaranteed her safety.

I told Debbie early on that I had read the police reports and was sorry to know that she had gone through such difficult experi-ences. "That's okay," she reassured me. "Not really," I responded. "Grown-up men should not have sex with children. That is *not* okay, it's against the law!" I remember her look of fascination when I first told her this. Eventually, "it's against the law" became the title of one of her poems. I also told her that I wished her mom could have taken better care of her and kept her safe. Debbie looked away. Throughout our therapy, she was loath to discuss her mother, exhibiting loyalty and empathy toward a mother few of us could understand. During my 43 years of working as a mental health professional, this was the first and only time I found it impossible to muster up any compassion for a mother who admitted to "encouraging them to pick the kid because she got more money that way." I'm sure that Debbie's mother had a long and painful history herself, but her responses to her daughter were beyond anything I had ever encountered, and I consider this type of maternal response quite rare. I pressed to have joint meetings with the mother and Debbie to gain some closure, especially when the mother's parental rights were terminated a year later. The mother refused, stating she didn't want anything to do with Debbie and that she had been "nothing but a pain in the ass" since the day she was born.

EARLY SESSIONS

Early sessions with Debbie focused on establishing trust, a tall order indeed. I made few demands of her, spoke plainly, and tried to be consistent and empathic (without any outward display of positive emotion that I suspected she might find so unfamiliar as to provoke further withdrawal). During some sessions, we listened to music that I asked her to bring in. She was very private about her drawings, but I hoped that one day she would draw or paint during our sessions. I showed her different things: She was very enthralled with "Butterfly Wisdom," a card game developed by a colleague of mine, Dr. Joyce Mills (Mills, 2007). In particular, she was taken with the notion that in order for the caterpillar to break out of its shell, it had to summon up some internal energy that was there from its birth, useful at a predetermined, specific moment that the caterpillar alone would sense. Because of her fascination with the idea of hidden energy that could become accessible, I gave her a present she cherished. There is a person who photographs butterflies from around the world without killing them to capture their beauty (Sandved, 1996). He finds letters of the alphabet on the wings and has a poster showing all the letters of the alphabet. In addition to ordering the poster, you can order a nameplate. I had asked her early on what name she wanted me to use, Deborah or Debbie. She said she preferred Aniston, her middle name. Whether she had been given a middle name was unclear, but she had taken one that she now wanted used. Thus, everyone who knew her called her Aniston, and since there were scant official records, some were created for her with this new name. I ordered a nameplate for her, and she cried holding it to her chest. She told me she now knew what a "prized possession" was.

Around the fourth month or so, I was feeling confident that the therapy relationship had grown stronger. I had met with her twice a week to increase the likelihood of her viewing therapy as reliable and consistent. During that time, I had not missed any appointments, even when one of them fell on a holiday. Her transportation was also perfectly constructed so that she always arrived a little early and left on time. She would sometimes see other youngsters leaving my room and asked about them. She always asked the same question: "Does that girl live with her mom?" She never inquired about boys. I answered that I couldn't say because of client confidentiality, and I told her that if they asked about her, I wouldn't say anything about her either. She seemed to accept my explanation, but I also asked her what she imagined about the girls and their moms. She would always respond that, yes, she thought the girls were living with their moms. In spite of her bleak childhood experiences, especially her relational foundation, it was great to see that this child was capable of imagining more positive caretaking for the peers she saw in my office. It also could have been an expression of longing for her mother, something I found bewildering but somewhat predictable in a grossly neglected child.

Aniston began to trust me. When she asked about other children coming to therapy that she saw in the waiting room, I had begun to make some statements that I hoped would make a dent in her defensive system. One day I told her about a 5-year-old who was missing her mother and hoping she could see her one day soon because her mother was sick and in the hospital. Another time I told Aniston about a boy whose father was "hooked on drugs" and was in a rehabilitation program. I also talked about a child who thought she was the cause of her dad beating her mom, and about another child who felt ashamed because her older brother had abused her sexually. This situation got her attention: "How old was her brother?"; "What did he do to her?"; "Do the kids at school know?"; and "Did he make her pregnant?" The last question surprised me, but I kept my responses steady and similar. She added, "They have to take it out and leak on the sheets so you don't get pregnant." She then confided, "Somebody told me that once, but I don't know who." I commented that she had learned things that most kids her age don't know about. She looked up and said, "I'm never doing that stuff again." I told her that was something she wouldn't have to think about again for a long, long time. She shook her head and said, "Uh, uh."

As we grew to know each other, I noticed that she looked more tired some days than others. She confided that she had "horrible, horrible nightmares" most nights, and she usually tried to stay awake to avoid dreaming. This lack of sleep began to take its toll, and when I talked to the teacher, she said as much about noticing Aniston's fatigue and lack of participation in the classroom. The teacher also said that Aniston had fallen asleep in the classroom on more than one occasion. When I asked about her academic standing, the teacher noted with surprise that she was catching up well and still keeping up, always doing a little more than expected. Aniston had confided that Sylvia, her teenage tutor, was "the best teacher," she had ever had.

When talking to the foster parents, they confirmed that it was hard to wake Aniston in the morning and that she was quite lethargic when she arrived home. They said that she liked being in her room most of the time and kept it tidy and well organized—behavior they had not seen in other foster children in their care.

During the first few months that I knew Aniston, she functioned well overall, but it seemed possible that her internalizing her traumatic experiences was causing her distress. She stayed mostly to herself, and trust continued to be an issue. Whenever she talked about her foster parents, she would say, "They're nice, but I'm not going to stay there very long." She seemed appropriately hesitant to get too attached to these temporary parents. During this time, her mother had been convicted of child endangerment and child neglect, sexual exploitation, and charges of trafficking, since she had moved her daughter over state lines to make her available to male clients. Aniston's social worker, who visited her twice a month, told me that Aniston's mother wanted nothing to do with her and would not object to termination of parental rights—she requested that her kid be "taken off her hands." Thus, we had kept Aniston informed of the parallel legal (criminal) process going on with her mother, and she likewise had expressed not caring.

ENCOURAGING POSTTRAUMATIC PLAY

I thought it was important for this child to begin to address her experiences and memories more directly so that she might have fewer nightmares and perhaps feel less compulsion to withdraw. I approached the topic directly with Aniston by telling her that I had brought some toys that I thought might help her show me a little bit about what it was like to live with her mother. I brought in a mother doll (with long black hair and provocative clothing like her mother) along with two other female dolls. I told her that I thought the figurine with the provocative clothing looked like her mom, but she could choose any of the three figures I brought for her to choose. She picked the same one I had picked. Then I gave her five smaller figurines of children and asked her to choose one to represent herself. She chose the smallest, the youngest one. Then I brought a bag full of men in different sizes, skin colors, and clothing. I didn't pour them out of the bag; instead, I had her pick the ones that looked like men she had met. She did so carefully and purposefully, and soon the cast of characters was chosen. I then gave her beds to choose from, small ones, big ones, beds with sheets, beds without. She took the mattress off one of the beds and said that most of the time she slept and "sexed" on the floor. She grabbed some cotton balls to use as pillows and said they were green. She asked for a marker and carefully painted each one green. "I used to like pillows," she volunteered. "They covered my head sometimes."

I took her to the dollhouse and told her that now that she had picked the cast of characters, she could now act like a movie director and show me a little about what it was like for her when her mother brought men to the house. "Just one, okay?" she said, and I said, "Sure." And so it went. She picked a room and put the mattress and green pillows on the floor. She put the little girl on the bed and put another bed next to hers. Then she grabbed the mother and showed her outside the house, standing, watching the cars go by. And she grabbed as many cars as she could and showed them going by.

The next sequence in this "scene" involved the mother grabbing one of the men and bringing him into the house. At the door she would say, "Me or her? Me or her?" Then Aniston would stop this play and ask to go to the bathroom. She almost always came back with a wet face which I saw as a good sign. Her thoughts and feelings were beginning to occur concurrently, and there was less compartmentalizing, although after she returned from the bathroom, she was not always eager to continue with the "movie." I had told her since the outset that it would be up to her when to start and stop since she was the director. It would also be up to her to show as much or as little as she wanted. This didn't seem problematic because when she got started, her scene took off and she was able to show details that were both shocking and remarkable. I had also given her a red card that she could pick up anytime to indicate that she wanted to stop the play, no questions asked. She used this card appropriately—not too often but enough to test its validity.

There were sessions when she would not reach for the bag in which she kept her figurines. I would notice this and would make explicit what she was doing. "I see that the director does not want to work today, and that's okay. All directors need breaks now and then." Other times the director came in the door eager to show different scenarios. Sometimes Aniston would say, "I remember somebody else," or "I remembered something else that happened." Each time I held my breath, nervous about what she would show me. And for the next 4 months or so, Aniston was in full posttraumatic play, re-creating scenes that she kept in her mind and that visited her in sleep. We took a picture of each session and wrote down some portion of the story told that day. We chronicled all that she remembered and felt. Early on, her stories were maintained at a distance. Aniston would talk about "the girl and her mother." As time went by, she began to talk about Aniston thinking or feeling something. We also incorporated Aniston's voice into her stories, at first by asking her to narrate what was going on and eventually asking her to give voice to the characters in her story. One session stuck in my mind for months. When the man walked out the door, the Aniston figurine yelled at her mother: "You didn't want me to be your kid; I don't want you to be my parent. You're nobody's parent."

Another session was also poignant. When Aniston brought one of the men to the room, he turned to the mother and yelled at her, "What? Are you crazy? She's only a kid. You're under arrest!!" The person who walked away was first a police officer but then became another little girl's father. "He's a good dad, like the one I live with now." Music to my ears. The foster father had followed every single directive I had given him about expressing positive interest in her from a distance. He had read her books at night in the living room, sitting on a chair opposite hers. He had been as patient and sweet as they come. I was already grieving the fact that this child would be moved to another home, but I hoped against hope for a good viable option for Aniston. I took great comfort in the fact that her adoption and placement worker was deeply invested in Aniston's future, and I worked closely with the case manager who had fallen in love with this child.

The posttraumatic play was not without stress. Aniston had full nights of being awake. She seemed fatigued and at times disoriented. She developed fresh symptoms of PTSD, especially emotionality and intrusive flashbacks. Luckily, she responded well to melatonin and was able to start sleeping again. She also became more verbal with me and her social worker. She still kept her distance from the foster parents, again saying, "They're nice, but I'm going to live somewhere else." I had weekly conversations with the parents who seemed concerned but began to see some subtle positive changes.

Slowly but surely, Aniston began to sleep better without melatonin and participated more fully at school. She had developed a friendship at school and talked about Mandy with great excitement. She liked sharing little things with her, like what she had for breakfast or a TV show she had watched. Mandy reciprocated and offered Aniston warmth and affection. One day she was ecstatic to report that Mandy's mom had taken her and Mandy to see a movie!

When she chose to engage with posttraumatic play, Aniston was relentless about documenting her memories and getting pictures that she took home. Unbeknownst to me or anyone else, she was filing the pictures in her journal and adding "ideas" about them prior to going to bed. It was as if she had successfully transferred her compartmentalizing abilities to the journal, closing it, and placing it inside a locked dresser drawer. Giving her a private place to store her private things was one of the best ideas the foster mother had.

The posttraumatic play provided a chronicle of this child's traumatic experiences, including some earlier memories of simply being left alone for days at a time. She couldn't remember anything prior to age 4 but imagined she "grew herself up" without help from anyone else.

One day she showed me a stunning piece of artwork that she had drawn in her journal—a hand that was reaching up toward the sun.

Her artwork spoke volumes about her spirit and her drive toward growth. She was never burdened by guilt or shame; she put those emotions squarely on the shoulders of her mother and the men who abused her. "I'm just a kid," she stated, "you're the grown-up, not me!"

Some important moments happened while I was still seeing her. She spontaneously ran into the arms of her foster father and hugged him. On that occasion, he surprised her by coming to pick her up (when he received a call that the transportation worker had taken ill). It was a moment I will not forget, and it happened well into the post-traumatic play and after she had faced what she had previously been unable to see, feel, or manage. Compartmentalization had served her well, but as she dismantled and laid out the layers of memories, it was clear that she was unburdening herself and becoming lighter.

During the play, we spent some time working on dissociation, which she called "my secret weapon." One day I found out how much she relied on dissociative responses when her green pillow got wet after her glass of water spilled over it. I said, "Oh, that's too bad, you usually put that on Aniston's head so she doesn't have to see." "That's okay," she told me, "I have my own secret weapon." When I asked about her secret weapon, she talked about "going away in her mind" and waking up when it was over. Like many child victims before her, she had learned to dissociate, to go away in her mind, to get away from the immediacy of her pain. She was shocked to learn that other kids do that when they are being hurt. She thought it was her very own creation; I confirmed that it was and that other kids had stumbled on the same secret weapons. I told her that she must have had lots of practice staying removed, inside herself, even when she was with other people. She smiled when I said that.

We ended up working a little on dissociation, especially her choosing it rather than having it "come on her" without her knowledge. We talked about when "going away" was a good idea and when it wasn't. I had her practice going away and coming back. Steadily, she became confident in her abilities to choose her own presence in different situations and with different people (Gil, 2006c).

The last momentous event that occurred in Aniston's life was her placement with an adoptive family. I met with them to help them think through what special needs they might need to support in Aniston, and I could not have picked a better family for her. They were attentive, kind, and, most of all, totally ready to adopt a child. As a bonus, they had a toddler at home, and their plan had always been to adopt a child after their own child was a toddler. The mother had had a high-risk pregnancy and would not be able to have another child. That news proved serendipitous because this couple had always planned to adopt. The first child they called their "miracle baby"; they dubbed Aniston their "second miracle child."

Aniston was appropriately sad to leave the first real home she'd ever known, and it was a tearful goodbye for us all. The only downside of the adoptive parents was that they lived three hours away, so Aniston would be referred to another therapist. The parents compromised and allowed an extended termination from this therapist. They brought her to me for therapy for about 9 months once a month. After that, I saw her quarterly for yet another year. Our therapy no longer included posttraumatic play. Instead, Aniston raised more age-appropriate concerns like sometimes wanting to be a baby like her little sister, getting in trouble with mom for "helping too much," and having small conflicts with a teacher who was not as patient as other teachers she had known. In therapy, she bathed and changed a babydoll's diapers. She absolutely loved the doll that she could feed and then would pee. My interpretation of this play was related to her observations of parenting in her new home as well as her longing to have had a normal infancy in which she was well cared for and nurtured and protected. She also brought pictures of her new room, her school, and her baby sister whom I had met once. She of course kept growing quickly, much to Aniston's pleasure and surprise at how quickly children grow.

This was one of the most rewarding experiences I have ever had as a therapist. It solidified my belief in children's resilience and in their amazing abilities to confront overwhelming traumatic experiences.

CONCLUSION

Many traumatized children naturally engage in posttraumatic play that they utilize at home, in other settings, and in the therapy environment. Shelby and Felix (2005) note that "the self-initiated posttraumatic play may be advantageous over therapist-directed posttraumatic play by providing the perception of increased control over content, pacing and mode of expression and exploration" (p. 84). However, some children, for whatever reason, are not able to access this reparative skill-set easily, and no matter how much time is afforded, or how many props are provided, it is impossible to facilitate posttraumatic play. In these situations, it becomes essential that clinicians make more directive and persistent clinical efforts to facilitate the emergence of posttraumatic play.

In my experience, the best clinical approach is to provide the child with objects that can be used literally and to manifest clinical confidence and a matter-of-fact style to communicate the expectation that children are capable of engaging in this work. Clinical conviction in the value and benefits of dynamic posttraumatic play is obviously an important requisite in presenting a positive therapeutic posture and conducting this type of therapy. Otherwise, clinical ambivalence, hesitation, or lack of conviction will be conveyed. In addition, those clinicians not experienced with helping children with unusual sexual knowledge will need to develop comfort so that they can engage in therapeutic curiosity and dialogue using developmentally appropriate terms.

This does not mean that clinicians need to be heavy-handed or rigid in their expectations. As our example with Aniston shows, she developed her own pacing and would often take breaks from the challenging processing involved in her posttraumatic play. Patience and respect, together with careful establishment of a solid therapy foundation (relationship), are important variables for this clinical intervention.

Posttraumatic play helps children organize their memories into concrete stories with beginnings, middles, and ends. As you saw with Aniston, she went from a passive victim stance to a more active experience of control over what she showed me (and what she showed herself), which of her insights she shared, and what statements she gave the characters to mutter. As children begin to use posttraumatic play, they may manifest symptoms and new behaviors that are concerning. It's important to anticipate an increase in problems as the play begins and also expect them to decrease over time. With time, Aniston had fewer nightmares, developed more trust in her foster parents, and opened herself up to new friendships. She became more outgoing as she developed more confidence in herself.

— *10* —

Burn Injuries

Danny was a slight, spunky little guy—a typical 6-year-old who seemed eager to come into the play therapy office and look around. His mother brought him to the intake session because Danny and his mother, Penny, were not used to separating too often. She seemed hypervigilant and anxious whenever she spoke about her son, and she hardly ever allowed him to be out of her sight. She talked about his social graces, his affability, his humor as well as her concerns about his acute startle response, his extreme fears of hurting himself, and his regression since an accident he had endured.

Danny had been at a friend's house when he inadvertently fell into a fireplace face forward, broke his fall with his arms, and incurred second-degree burns on his hands, arms, and chest. He had been hospitalized in the burn unit for 6 weeks and had been home for about a couple of months when she brought him to therapy.

Penny, a single mother, talked about Danny's adjustment, which mostly sounded good; however, it appeared to me that he was struggling with signs of PTSD (especially emotionality and anxiety) and seemed to require a great deal of comforting and reassurance. Penny wondered if the changes in Danny's personality would persist and kept repeating that she "just wanted her little boy back." It was evident that she felt very guilty about the accident, starting with letting him have a play date alone. She told me that she usually stayed at his play dates and didn't allow her son to go overnight to anyone's house. When I took a developmental history during intake, many things fell

135

into place: Her significant vigilance preceded the accident and somehow strengthened her resolve to watch her growing son to the best of her ability. Penny repeated that this was her "one and only" because her doctors had told her she would never become pregnant again. She described a highly difficult pregnancy, with Danny being a premature child, born with a congenital heart defect that required surgery when he was 3 weeks old. He had subsequent surgeries at 2 and 4 years of age and would likely need another surgery in the near future. His vulnerabilities and early hospitalizations had likely caused Penny's grave concern about her son. She said he had been in therapy before, when he was 4, but his therapist had moved to another state. (Eventually, when I communicated with Danny's previous therapist, she remarked that "mother is fiercely protective of her son, sometimes to the detriment of his development.")

I told Penny that I would see Danny in individual therapy to work on the trauma of his accident, and I also alerted her that I wanted to see him alone as soon as he was comfortable separating from her. I told her that, in addition, there would be times when I would ask her into the session for conjoint sessions since the accident had happened to them both and they had both suffered the consequences in different ways. Mother was on board with treatment to focus on traumatic impact but worried that he wouldn't be able to tolerate her being out of the room. My initial impression was that it would be the mother who would need to build a tolerance to letting her son stay in session without her.

BEGINNING THERAPY

Danny was a delight, full of energy and curiosity. Initially, his attention was unfocused as he explored drawing, painting, building, playing with cars, and setting up gladiator fights with the castle. The king was a significant toy for him, and he often yelled out orders to his men, giving himself a strong, authoritative voice. I wondered who his male role models were and how he understood not having a father figure in his life. Mother had only said that she had never been interested in romantic relationships and always knew she would be a single mother. I made a mental note to ask her how she had explained this to her boy.

From the outset, Danny showed interest in the dolls, boy and girl dolls equally. Coincidentally, one of our dolls has a scar drawn on its chest, drawn by a child who had open-heart surgery. This doll also has a gauze bandage on its arm, placed there by another child. All the therapists using the office decided to leave the gauze on the doll, and so we did. Some children were very drawn to the "injured child" doll. Initially, Danny avoided the injured doll but later on, used it to start a phase of focused play that would become useful to him.

I began to observe that Penny had a range of uncomfortable reactions to Danny's play and would mostly cue him nonverbally. Sometimes she would gasp, grunt, or use a variety of "hmms." Other times she would stand up quickly, come toward him, stand behind him, or lean forward. She gave very few verbal directives, although she would offer a few "Be careful" and "Watch out" statements as Danny exhibited more energy. One particular theme emerged overtly: any time Danny used his hands and arms, his mother would slow him down or pull him back from his activity. Thus, when he attempted to throw the darts at the target, she would say, "Let's not do that today." When Danny wanted to swing a nerf bat to strike a ball, she would take the bat out of his hands and ask him to find something else to do. Danny always complied. Penny told me that his burns were mostly healed but added that, to avoid pain, he had been cautioned about making too many broad movements. She still had a regimen to prevent infection in some of his burned areas. It's important to note that Danny's burns were not minor. He never showed me his chest burns, but his hands were quite obviously burned, although he didn't show any signs of self-consciousness. His movement seemed impaired at times but not too often. Danny never talked about pain during our sessions, but it became clear that he had suffered a lot during the burn treatments.

After a few months, I had to nudge Penny about leaving the session. I usually tell parents to say they're going to the bathroom and then just take a long break, eventually not returning. Mother took very small breaks, always returned, and I had to ask her to sit in the waiting room. Since it seemed so difficult to her, I told Danny that his mom would be waiting outside for him. He didn't blink an eye, which caused Penny to ask him if it was okay and to give him a long hug and ask him to come get her if anything happened. (It was very important to coach her and help her realize that her anticipating problems was contributing to some of Danny's difficulties.)

POSTTRAUMATIC PLAY

Danny's posttraumatic play began in earnest at about the fifth month when he resumed focused attention on the boy doll. To this point, my approach had been nondirective, and it appeared to me that Danny was quite responsive to a permissive environment, one in which he could direct his play, set his own limits, and express himself more openly. I had learned a lot about him, especially by seeing the contrast between his individual and joint sessions. The parent–child dynamic would require attention since Danny was adapting his behavior to his mother's spoken and unspoken anxiety about his safety.

At first, Danny picked up the doll and seemed to want approval from me to play with it. I made simple statements such as "You keep going back to check out that doll," or "You are checking him out head to toe." He would always respond, "It's a boy!" I never judged his choosing the doll, and I never encouraged or discouraged it. I also never interpreted that he liked or seemed interested in the doll, I simply described his behavior. The child-centered approach worked best for Danny at this juncture.

His interest in the boy doll became continuous as he would always pick it up early in the sessions, placing it on the desk (calling it a "table"). He undressed the doll and then used the stethoscope to listen to the doll's heart. Often he would shift his attention to my heart and his own. He counted both my heartbeat and his. Once I asked him to listen to his heart after he had run to the bathroom and back. He enjoyed knowing his heart could get fast and slow.

When he asked for a "gown" for the doll, I ordered a big shirt for it. He also asked that it tie on the back. I sewed some little strings on the back of the shirt and cut it open. He smiled widely when he saw the "gown." Then he asked me to buy some sticky Band-Aids. We had some circular Band-Aids in the office, but he wanted the long ones. Once I got them, he asked for bigger, white tape. I returned to the drug store for white tape and gauze. Danny was very appreciative and quickly began cutting and taping, cutting and taping. He always taped up the top part of the doll, leaving the legs exposed. Then he would pull off the tape, all the while saying, "Breathe, breathe." After this routine, he would take some cream and massage the child on his head, making small circles on the head, forehead, and sinus areas. When Danny engaged in this play, he looked to be in a trance. His body was still. His breaths were shallow. When he told the doll to breathe, I would take a long, loud inhale and exhale. A couple of times, he smiled when I exhaled and he took a deep breath himself.

He began talking to the doll regularly. "How are you feeling this morning?" he would ask, or "Can I get anything for you?" He wanted to make a buzzer for his doll so that he could ring for the nurses. I brought in the buzzer from a game I had at home ("Taboo"), and he was thrilled. When the batteries ran low, he had a tear in his eyes. "It's broken," he said. I told him it was just low on batteries, and I would bring some in for it. Danny spontaneously hugged me when I remembered to bring in the batteries for his buzzer.

There were sessions in which Danny bathed his doll, letting him soak in very long baths. During those times, he would play with other things, going back to check on the doll over and over, "Is the water comfortable?" Danny kept the buzzer nearby, and he would tell the doll, "Remember, you can call if you need anything." The doll would buzz frequently at first, but then he stopped doing so. One time, the doll buzzed and then laughed when the nurse came (that would be me). He had instructed me to say, "Everything okay?" The doll said, "Yup, just wanted to see if your hair was the same color." This was a reference to the fact that I had changed my hair color. Few people noticed, but Danny was a skilled observer.

When Danny pulled the tape off, he began to whimper. "I notice you're making little sounds," I said, to which he responded, "This hurts a lot!" I told him I was sorry it hurt a lot. The whimpers became louder and louder until one day he "burst open" how much it hurt and made a long, loud yell. He actually held out his arms, took a deep breath, and yelled at the top of his lungs. He then took a few steps toward me and repeated the motion. I did not move, even though it was pretty loud. "Wow," I said, "you have a very loud yell to show how big your pain is." He seemed surprised; he backed up and said "My mom doesn't like it when I screamed." Serendipity—his mother was at the door. "Is he okay?" "Oh yes," I reassured her, "he's doing just fine." She asked if she "should" come in, and I told her it was not necessary. When I returned to Danny, he no longer wanted to play and moved on to dressing the boy doll with some other clothes.

My educated guess is that this play lasted about 12 consecutive sessions, and it was at this point that Penny made an appointment to tell me she was concerned that her son was "regressing." When I asked her to describe what was going on, she mentioned that Danny was isolating himself in his room, seemed irritable, even angry at her, and would not sleep in his bed alone. She also mentioned that he was crying at the drop of a hat, even when he just bumped into the corner of a table. Mother's anxiety was heightened, and she sounded angry as she complained that I was "keeping things from her" and that I seemed "reluctant to share information about his treatment." I told her that I was sorry that she had that impression and reviewed his progress (yet again). But hearing that his play was on target, that he was using play in a very useful way, and that he was obviously work-ing out some of the trauma of his stay in the hospital for the burns did not calm her in any way. "This is what I mean, you never say anything specific: What is he saying, what kind of play is he doing, why does he scream in your office?" I tried again to give her some information while respecting Danny's confidentiality. Finally, I told her that as soon as it was possible, I would have her come into ther-apy with Danny, and he could show her himself the kind of work he was doing. Danny had told me twice that he liked keeping his mother out of our sessions. The following week, after she came to the door asking about why he was yelling, Danny, slowly but surely, pushed a chair in front of the door.

Danny's play started to become less focused. During the last phase of the play, he often asked questions: "Can this child resume normal activity?" Huh? I was taken aback by the adult language. "Will his heart be able to endure? Will he live a normal life now?" I could only assume that he had heard his mother ask the doctors these questions. Sometimes he would answer the questions himself. Other times he would almost whisper, "We just don't know what impact this will have long term." It became clear that Danny likely worried about his general health and his fortitude.

Danny's doll remained in his clothes most of the time now, his gown neatly folded and placed under a pillow in the crib. He took the doll out of the crib and kept him out most of the time. If someone else had played with it and put it back in the crib, he would take it out. He started hiding the doll when he left, and I left it where Danny placed it. The first time he returned to find it hidden, he said, "Ha, ha, that was a good hiding place!" "I see that," I noted. Toward the end of his play, he dubbed his doll "Arson."

It seemed that the posttraumatic play had caused some relief as well as some regression. Overall, I felt that Danny had done what he needed to do with the memories of being in the hospital and the release of his silent screams of pain. He had also nurtured the boy doll through his injuries and taken great care to feed him, check his vitals, and encourage him to walk and talk to friends. Throughout, he was purposeful, in and out of trance, and in complete control of where he took his story. Now the conjoint family work could begin.

CONJOINT SESSIONS

At first, Danny was not pleased with the idea of conjoint sessions. He asked if his mother *had* to come in or if we could go to another room, not his room. He asked what he would have to talk about with his mom. He asked if he had to show her Arson, the doll. I wondered what it would be like for him to show mom Arson. Danny was adamant: "She'll ask him a ton of questions and drive him crazy!!" When I inquired how Arson would feel about being asked a lot of questions, he said, "What do you think?" He was definitely not happy with me.

I reassured him that he could spend time with her doing whatever he wanted. It was up to him what he showed her and what they did together. "Fine," he said, "let's make her paint!" True to form, he asked to go into the art therapy office, and he and his mom undertook a painting project. While his mom suggested they share the large piece of paper, he signaled me to put up the other easel, which I did. They each had their own piece of paper, and they picked their own paints and brushes. Danny was downright surly, and I was interested to see how they would work things out. Mother took control early, asking Danny to make a picture of a dog. "NO, I don't want to!" Mom pleaded with him and then stated that *she* would make the dog instead. Penny had some good artistic skills and kept talking about the mistakes she made; she erased a lot and kept trying to make it look perfect. I said nothing and chose instead to watch their interaction. As soon as Danny started to draw a picture of a large tree, his mother gave a long list of directives: "Don't make it too big for the page, make sure it's a fall tree," "Try to use different colors for the leaves," and "Stand close to the easel so you don't have to stretch your arms so much." As this process continued and the hour drew to a close, both seemed frustrated and disappointed with what they had done. "I'm not too sure drawing is my specialty area," Penny said. Danny looked at me on the way out and said, "Thanks for nothing."

We had about six more sessions like this, but my observations were invaluable. The patterns of interaction were on display in each session, some more than others. By the second session, Penny asked: "When are we going to deal with some of the real issues going on?" I anticipated this question and reminded her that things take time. "I know," she said, "but how long?" She hated the response I gave her: "As long as it takes for him to feel comfortable enough to share." Later I met with her alone and asked her what she had noticed about the sessions. She answered that there wasn't anything "new" going on. "I guess you're seeing exactly what I deal with at home. He used to be really sweet and easygoing; now he stomps his feet, he's combative, and he wants to stay by himself a lot." I commented that I had noticed her frustration with his not following her lead, and I asked her to consider laying back, letting him take the lead or allowing him to play in any way he wanted, without any directive from her. She didn't like the suggestion, stating that if she did that, "nothing would get done." I told her that her backing up would allow him to fill up the space more, to lead himself, to be more himself. She was skeptical but finally agreed, stating: "I don't know that I can be as passive as you." I let that comment go and just asked her to give it a try.

Danny noticed the change in his mother and was provocative with her. "Why are you being so weird?" Penny looked at me for an answer. I didn't respond. Slowly but surely, Danny began to explore the room and interact with me as if his mother wasn't there. I thought this was a sign of progress, although Penny initially took offense and told her son he was being rude.

Penny leaned into being "passive" as she called it and responded well to writing down her observations about Danny's play in therapy. Suddenly, their dynamic had changed; they were in the same room, and there was little conflict. Danny would take things to show his mother; he would turn and ask her questions. I had instructed her to simply validate and not talk too much. She had told me how difficult this was for her but noticed that the less she said, the more her son volunteered information. She bought herself a journal and wrote down 10 to 15 pages after each session. We met weekly, and I listened to her insights, questions, and worries.

Ever so slowly, Danny took Arson out of the crib and showed it to his mother with two other dolls. Subsequently, he showed her the "gown" I had sewn for the doll. Eventually, he showed his mother how he taped Arson up, took his blood pressure, gave him baths, and kept inquiring if he needed anything. I noticed his reluctance to show his mother any evidence of pain. I thought I would facilitate Danny's release of this aspect of the play in some way. When he asked me to be the nurse, I asked the usual questions that he had prompted me to say. But on this one occasion, I added, "Can I get you anything for the pain?" He looked at me quizzically. "I didn't say he hurt." I stayed in the nurse role and said, "All children who have burn treatments have a lot of pain, and sometimes they cry softly or loudly." He glanced over at his mother. I nodded to her, and she repeated what I had just said, "That's right little boy. We can get you something for the pain; it's okay to show that something hurts." I believe that might have been the first time Danny heard this from his mom. She had told me that she usually told him, "Everything will be fine," or "It's almost over," but she never acknowledged the pain. In one of our conversations, Penny had confided that when her infant son was in the intensive care unit, she "pretended" that he did not feel any pain because his nerves were still underdeveloped. "This was my best coping strategy, to pretend he could feel no pain, and to tell myself that he would not remember anything about this."

Danny didn't respond but stopped the play and went over to stand next to his mother. Sometimes they looked downright uncomfortable with each other. "He might be needing a hug," I said to Penny, and she reached out to hug him. "Are you okay?" she asked, "Is this too tight?" Danny let go and moved back to see me. "What time is it?" he asked. He had obviously had his fill, so we stopped a little early.

After this session, Arson went missing in action in front of his mother. However, when we met individually, Arson took center stage. Danny always stopped at the same place in the play, the place where Arson would yell out his pain. I wondered whether his reluctance was that he worried that others would hear him, as his mother had. I invited them to come with me to the back of the building, and I told Danny that I thought he might like the experience of yelling as loud as he wanted and knowing that his yell would go into the outside and his mother could hear him without worry. He asked me to yell first, and I did. He waited to see if anyone would come, and no one did. Danny then bent over, breathed in, and stood up, yelling at the top of his lungs. "Wow," I said, "that was a big one." Two other yells followed. His mother also expressed her pride at his good lungs. "I thought you might be wanting to yell somewhere where you didn't have to worry about other people. "That's cool," he said. I put a little seed in his mind, "Everyone likes to yell out without worry; I bet even your mom would like that." He left chewing on that statement.

His mother called me midweek to tell me that Danny had pulled her by the hand and they had gone outside, to their back yard. There he showed her how loud he could be and asked her to show how loud she could be. Apparently, he enjoyed himself with his mother.

The next session, I again decided to take the lead, and midway in the session, I told Danny that I was going to get Arson out. He did not object. I then told Danny that his mom wanted to talk to Arson and tell him something important. Mother repeated exactly what we had rehearsed on the phone, and I paraphrase here:

> Little boy, I wanted to tell you something very important. It was very hard for me to see you in pain. I cried a lot about your pain. If I had been able to trade places with you and take away your pain, I would have. I was so scared for you, scared how I would help you get past your horrible pain. So I think I hurried you, told you it would pass soon, tried to distract you. But I forgot to tell you that I knew you were in pain, that I was sorry you were in pain, and that it was okay to cry and yell and do whatever you wanted to do to show your pain. I'm sorry that I told you to be quiet, and told you to be brave. You are only little, you were

scared, and you can always count on your mom to love you and help you feel better.

To say that Danny melted is an understatement. I could see his eyes tear. However, I had instructed Penny to talk to Arson and not to Danny and to let Danny come to her. Danny did not. He took his time to let this information sink in.

Penny reported that the week following this session was "plainly remarkable." She talked about how he asked her to read a story, wanted her to stay with him until he fell asleep, slept in his own bed, and, most importantly, seemed like his old self, happy and easygoing. She told me she was afraid "for the other shoe to drop" but hoped against hope that the changes would continue, and they did, for the most part.

I structured termination with Danny over a period of time. He was not happy to leave therapy but understood that it was time for him to stop coming. His mother was providing consistent and empathic care, and her hypervigilance had decreased significantly. During her observations of the play therapy sessions, she had discovered that her son did better when he was treated as if he was a strong and capable young child. She had insights about how afraid she had been about his heart condition as well as a full recovery from the burns. She realized that she needed some help to continue to "let go" of the past, and I urged her to see her own psychotherapist. She had wanted to come see me, but I thought it might concern Danny to terminate therapy and know his mother was continuing. Penny established a very good connection with her therapist, and this mother–son dyad made great strides.

CONCLUSION

Danny had some early medical challenges and had shown himself to be a rugged little fighter. Penny was a loving and protective mother who had developed a great deal of anxiety in response to her infant child's heart condition, which had required several hospitalizations. She had coped by imagining that her son did not feel pain and by distracting him from overt expression of pain. When Danny had a terrible accident in which he suffered second-degree burns on his hands, arms, and chest, his mother felt burdened by guilt for not having protected him sufficiently. Guilt and anxiety created an emotional climate for Danny's recovery, especially his ongoing needs for nurturing caretaking. While Penny followed every recommendation to ensure Danny's progress, she inadvertently treated Danny as if he was more fragile than he really was. In addition, although burn treatment is very painful, she had not facilitated Danny's release of pain. Thus, he had silenced his crying and his screams.

The burn treatment was very hard on Danny, compounded by his mother's specific responses to him. Thus, posttraumatic play allowed him to externalize and resolve some of the embedded conflicts that had occurred during his recovery. The issues were intrapsychic as well as systemic, so his therapy consisted of both individual and family therapy sessions. A significant theme emerged when Danny gave the doll the opportunity to yell and release his pain. Giving voice to the pain he had suffered seemed like an important abreactive experience for Danny. Sharing that experience with his mother further reinforced the importance of releasing affect, especially to someone he loved but felt distress when he expressed his pain.

This case demonstrates the importance of allowing children to play out unresolved traumatic experiences and doing so within the child's familial context. In addition, this mother did a tremendous amount of work on herself and accepted my recommendations for her to behave in ways that were counterintuitive for her. This case demonstrates, once again, that taking the time to build therapeutic trust with both the child and his mother pays off in spades.

— *11* —

Chronic Sexual Abuse

*B*etsy was a 9-year-old with an extensive history of sexual abuse, starting at approximately 3 years of age. She was removed twice from her mother, Laura, who failed six different rehabilitation programs. Laura had been raised in the foster care system and was quite young with her own history of abuse. Unfortunately, Laura was herself a highly traumatized woman who was unable to make use of the ample services that had been provided to her. When I met Betsy, Laura's parental rights had been terminated, and she was in yet another rehabilitation program. Betsy's father had been incarcerated for most of her young life, convicted on charges of aggravated assault, attempted murder, and sexual abuse of a minor. Betsy had experienced sexual abuse at his hands and the hands of his friends, and yet she stood before me, a sweet, happy, carefree little girl—at least that's how she seemed at first. She had been in a foster care placement for nearly 9 months before coming to therapy. She had been to a pediatrician, a dentist, and an optometrist, all in the first 6 months of this placement—some of her teeth had been pulled, her diet had been changed, and she had close monitoring by her pediatrician. She had reportedly been a sickly child, but because she had not formally entered schools, immunization records had not been requested or collected. Laura had always kept Betsy with her, even when they were homeless on the street, and they had both been in homeless shelters together. When sober, Laura was very receptive to services and quite loving to her child. Betsy's social worker did everything in her power to ensure that Laura received as much help as possible and prioritized Betsy's needs for safety, stability, and education. Betsy loved her mother and asked after her frequently, but she thrived in the foster home with a single foster mother, Miss Mary, who worked as a part-time school counselor. Betsy was aware that she would likely move somewhere else and remained cordial and polite with Mary. I suspected that Betsy was unwilling to make too much of an investment, especially because she believed that most people in her life eventually left.

Betsy had ostensibly understood that her mother's termination of parental rights was a permanent decision by the judge. Laura had explained to her daughter that she was unable to care for her as she deserved. Laura also made clear that she was the one with the problem, not Betsy. They had cried together as Laura explained her drug addiction, her inability to get or keep a job, and the fact that Betsy should be studying regularly in school and should have a family who could take better care of her. During their goodbye session, Laura had asked Betsy to forgive her for all the times she left her alone, for not protecting her from her father, and for being asleep when she should have been awake. Of course, Betsy remembered some of the frightening experiences they had endured, but she had always been protective of her mother and asked Laura what her plans were for herself. Laura was able to tell her that she was going to go to a rehabilitation program yet again and continue to try to get over her addiction, make better choices, and maybe even go to school herself one day. The social worker told me that in that goodbye meeting, the mother–daughter role reversal was very much on display. Betsy reassured her mother and eventually wished her well. Laura asked few questions about Betsy's life, and Betsy volunteered little information to her mother. She did tell her mother, however, that Miss Mary was helping her a lot and that she was happy where she was.

BEGINNING THERAPY

When I first met Betsy, she appeared quite capable and mature. She responded well to my review of what therapy was and what I knew about her. She told me that when she was "a lot younger" she had been to see a therapist for "a little while," but she didn't remember when or where. When I asked about her previous therapy, she was unable to say much about what she liked, what issues had been addressed, or what the therapist was like or even what he or she looked like. She did remember that the therapist had long blond hair and that she liked to play cards with her.

Betsy explored the room freely and touched and played with many of the toys and activities in the room. As a few sessions went by, she seemed intrigued by the order of the toys and liked noticing that things were still in their place, precisely where she had left them the week before. She didn't use a routine of any kind, as many children do. She started with different activities each time, played briefly with this and that, and then moved on to something else. Her play was not necessarily creative, but rather, she used concrete or literal symbols. For example, when she did a play genogram and I invited her to choose a miniature that best showed her thoughts or feelings about everyone in the family, including herself, she chose a lock and key for her father, a bottle of wine and cigarettes for her mother, and a school girl for herself. When I asked her to find something to represent her current foster mother, Miss Mary, she picked a Bible because Miss Mary "prays every night." I encouraged her to find some other things, but she couldn't think of anything else. When I asked if there were any other important people in her life, she couldn't think of any.

When I asked her to draw or color, Betsy usually drew a sky, with a sun and clouds. She almost always made a ground line with flowers coming out of a grassy area. She never drew a house or a person, even when I invited her to make a self-portrait or make a picture of the house where she currently lived. When she did not want to comply, she simply shrugged her shoulders.

I also invited her to do a collage about what it was like for her in school. She found it nearly impossible to find pictures that she thought would be relevant, although she did find a lunch box and then cut out a picture of an apple as well as a bottle of milk.

She played some in the sandbox but without miniatures and without telling or showing stories. She usually used her hands in the sand and repeated how soft and clean the sand was. She kept the sand dry, although a few times she asked if it would be okay to wet the sand. I told her it was okay to use the water, but she never ventured out of her comfort zone.

My impression of Betsy was that she was emotionally constricted, an observer of life who was not able to fully trust enough to let go of her inhibitions. Sometimes it appeared that she wasn't used to being visible to this clinician. Other times, she whispered to make sure that I would ask what she was saying. It was almost as if she were used to being compliant and following others' rules. It was hard for her to assert her needs or wants, at least in the therapy setting. When I used child-centered play therapy, she was acutely uncomfortable. I remember her asking, "Why do you repeat what I say?" and "Why do you talk so funny?" Eventually, I decreased the number of reflective statements I made and acquiesced to her wanting me to lead the way. When I asked her to participate in different activities, she did so readily. One of the activities was to make a list of things she might want to do during our sessions. She could not think of anything. When I asked her what we had already done that she enjoyed enough to repeat, she couldn't think of anything. When I asked her if there was something at school she enjoyed, she couldn't think of a thing, and when I asked about Miss Mary, she offered that she liked having picnics with her in their back yard. That was something I told her we could do in back of our office one day. (When we did, she enjoyed going outside but seemed very matter of fact about the menu.)

Betsy was an enigma: She had suffered chronic and severe abuse most of her life, and she had recently lost the only parent she had. And yet she carried on, doing what she was supposed to do, catching up academically, and adjusting to her new environment, even though it was the polar extreme of what she had known with her mother. She did not seem to have overt symptoms of distress, and as I said before, she rolled with the punches, made the best of things, and got along with her foster mother and her teachers. She didn't have any special friendship, but it seemed her peers at school included her in their play at recess, and she was happy to interact with them and follow their lead. This child was very resilient, and she had learned to simply fit in, in order to survive. My guess is that given her mother's erratic behavior and instability, she had developed a matter-of-fact attitude about the experiences she had and the encounters with strange or dangerous people. A lot was expected of her from an early age, and she rose to every occasion, raising herself in a way, learning to self-soothe and regulate herself. She organized her resources to take care of her mother, and when her mother spent time away from home, Betsy simply waited, entertaining herself by watching television. She eventually confided that she liked to find hiding places no matter where she was. She also showed me the part of my room that she had zeroed in on the first time she came in. She was certain that she could fit behind one of the couches if she laid down very flat and very straight. I was amazed to hear that she had identified a hiding place on her first visit. She had a quiet, confident way of fending for herself. I am always in awe of what children can do not just to survive but to thrive in very unfriendly, stark, or chaotic environments.

Thus, our first 6 months of therapy proceeded in this fashion. I could say that we were getting to know each other, but in truth, I never felt emotionally connected to this child during this time, and I was often mystified about what she was doing or about the benefit of what was happening in therapy. Amazingly, in about the fourth month, Miss Mary called to tell me that Betsy was sick with a cold but was crying because she wanted to come to therapy "no matter what." Miss Mary had agreed to call me and check to see if it was okay if the child came even though she had a little cold. I was shocked. I had no idea that therapy had any particular meaning for Betsy, and of course I told her to go ahead and come but to bring lots of tissues.

Betsy's life had been full of unexpected changes, and at the sixth month, a most amazing turnaround occurred: Social services had identified and approached one of Betsy's aunts who, miraculously, lived in a nearby county. The aunt and mother had been estranged all their lives. This aunt, Estela, had also been in foster care at some point in her early life; however, unlike her sister Laura, she had special medical needs, so she had been placed for adoption when she was 4 and Laura was 7. How Estela was located was a mystery the social worker could not share with me, but suddenly there was a viable option of a blood family member who might be willing to consider adopting this child. Estela was married, divorced, and widowed, and raising twin girls who were currently 14 years old. Serendipity— Estela was receptive to meeting her niece and saddened to hear about Laura's trajectory in life. A meeting was arranged, and I met with Estela prior to her meeting Betsy. To say I was impressed with Estela is an understatement. She was a woman in her early 40s whose husband had been killed in Iraq. She was a financial consultant and worked out of her home. She lived in a small but comfortable house, and her children went to a local public high school. She described a strong bond to her adoptive parents and was grateful they had provided her with a wonderful home and solid values. She described her childhood as happy and "full of love." She noted that she had been born with a congenital heart defect and needed several operations when she was young. She was now in good health, followed a strict diet and exercise regimen, and felt very fortunate to live in an era in which medical care is sophisticated and advanced. Her twins had been normal births, and neither had any medical concerns. She described her own happy family and noted that her husband's death was devastating to all three. The 4-year anniversary of his death was coming up shortly.

Estela asked few questions about Betsy and had been informed of Betsy's childhood by the social worker. She was full of questions about Laura, however. The social worker had given her Laura's last known address, but Laura had already left that address (she left the rehab center prematurely) and her present whereabouts were unknown. The social worker said that Laura had a friend on the West Coast, and she was thinking of going there in the future. Estela was disappointed that she might not ever see her older sister again and seemed to have some positive memories of her.

I prepared Estela the best I could to meet Betsy, and true to form Betsy was matter of fact about the meeting. She was pleasant and respectful to her aunt and showed her around the office. At times like this, Betsy seemed much older than her 9 years. Betsy invited Estela to play a game of cards, and Estela seemed content to do whatever Betsy wanted to do. Their meeting went well, as I knew it would, and they arranged for Betsy to come for the weekend to meet her cousins. The social worker arranged the logistics of this visit, and when I saw Betsy the following week, she was full of stories about her cousins. She said they were "identical twins," and she knew which was which because "one has long hair and the other short!" She said their house was really nice, and there was a room just for her. When Miss Mary came to get her that day, Betsy said she could have stayed longer with me. This was the most enthusiasm I had ever seen from this child.

Over the following months, the visits continued to go well, and hopes were high among the professionals working on this case (myself, the social worker, and the guardian ad litem [a child's attorney]) that Estela might adopt the child. One day Estela asked to speak to me and said she had one concern, and that was that Betsy had made some inappropriate comments to her daughters. While she thought the girls had handled it well, she wanted to know if this was normal for Betsy and what more she could expect. I asked her what specifically had happened, and she was a little shy to report that Betsy had asked one of the twins a question about one of the twins' boyfriend. "He's cute. Do you have to suck his dick?" Marlene, Betsy's cousin, had said to her, "We don't use that kind of language, Betsy," and walked away to consult with her mother. After doing so, she came back to Betsy and said, "Betsy, I know you've learned some things in your life about sex, but the things that happened to you should never have happened to a little kid. Whoever touched you or made you touch them was wrong to do that." "I already know that," Betsy responded and walked away, looking both a little irritated and a little embarrassed. I talked to Estela about sexual abuse and told her that the fact that Betsy was bringing this up was a good sign. I also told her that chances were that seeing her twin cousins with their boyfriends (couples) was likely triggering memories of male–female relationships. Estela noted that Betsy had seen one of her cousins kissing her boyfriend, and Estela had reprimanded her, cautioning her to be super careful about public displays of affection. When I heard this, however, I thought it was time to attempt more directive work with Betsy about her sexual abuse. I did not want anything to ruin her chances of being adopted by her aunt. In addition, I felt that the first phase of our work together had solidified: Betsy was comfortable with me and seemed to trust that she was safe in my presence. The fact that Miss Mary was a solid attachment figure in her life also served her well. I think Betsy was beginning to believe that life could be predictable and stable and that there were people whom she could turn to with questions.

POSTTRAUMATIC PLAY

I asked Estela to tell Betsy that she had told me about the statement she had made to her cousin Marlene and how Marlene had responded.

When Betsy came in at the next session, I told her that Estela had talked to me about what she had said to her cousin. Instead of asking questions, I simply said, "I agree with Marlene that what happened to you should not happen to any child." Betsy looked quizzically and asked how I knew what had happened to her when she was little. I asked her to think back to when we first started meeting and reminded her that her social worker had given me information about all the things that had happened to her when she was young. "But she doesn't know everything," Betsy said, "I never told her." "I'm sure it's been hard to tell anyone about what happened" I said softly, "but just because you don't talk about it, doesn't mean it's not there." "Yeah," she said, "but I don't like talking about it because it's gross!" "I'm sure you think of it as gross," I responded. "To me what's gross is that grown-ups can think to hurt kids that way." "Nothing really hurt," she said, "it was just gross."

And so the conversation began with many long, avoidant pauses. I thought it best to begin a project and used the Color Your Life technique by Kevin O'Connor (Hall, Kaduson, & Schaefer, 2002). To start, however, I asked her to make a list of "feelings you have most of the time" and then to pick a color that best showed the feeling. She filled in little boxes next to the feelings, and she chose: *worried,* orange; *sad,* blue; *numb,* gray; *happy,* yellow. I told her she could add other feelings at any time. After she finished making this list and assigning colors, I asked her to use these colors to paint her life so far. I made a horizontal line and put birth on one end and 9 years old at the other. I extended the line to 18 at one point. Using the colors she had assigned, she began to color the line with the feelings she had when she was little and older, and she added "afraid" to the list and chose the color purple. Her Color Your Life drawing included purple (afraid) and orange (worried) until she was about 6. At that time she added gray and more orange. Her final removal from her mother had occurred when she was 7, so at 7 years her colors were blue (sad) and gray (numb). I asked her what color she felt now, and she added orange (worried). I extended the line a little and asked her about her feelings, and she said, "You mean, if I stay with Miss Mary, or if I go with my Aunt Estela?" I told her we could make both lines because we didn't really know. She added yellow (happy) at the line for her life with Estela and put in Marlene and Charlene's names as well.

I asked her when she had felt the most afraid in her life, and she marked around 5 or 6. When I asked what was happening that scared her so much, she answered, "My dad was doing bad things." This was the opening I had hoped for to help her process the sexual abuse experiences.

Eventually, she was able to make a "secret list" of what her father had done. It looked like extensive sexual abuse by her father and other men. When I asked who the other men were, she said "friends of my dad who drank a lot of beer." Whenever I could I would state how sorry I was this had happened to her and how angry I felt that these men would think to do these things. "People who touch children's private parts have a problem in the way they think and feel. They make bad choices, and they need help to stop hurting children. This makes me really sorry for you that this happened and really mad that men think they can hurt children like this," I would say firmly. Eventually, she said: "Me too!" But at first she seemed surprised by my reaction.

One day I asked her to make a picture of anything she remembered about the abuse. She made six oblong shapes on the page with a firm, thick black marker. "That's what I remember," she said, "dicks and more dicks." "Dicks and more dicks," I repeated, feeling uncomfortable with the word. "Yep, dicks everywhere." She made the penises standing up, but I noticed some were horizontal. "They sleep, they wake up, they sleep, they wake up." "You've met a lot of dicks," I said, "sleeping ones and ones that were awake." "It's gross," she repeated, and proceeded to cover the page with big lines until the penises were not visible.

What followed was an exploration of this little girl's experiences with adult males who exploited and misused her for their sick entertainment. To spare the reader vicarious traumatization, I will spare the details here. Suffice to say, this child had survived tremendous abuse at the hands of her father and a group of his friends (all now imprisoned for their crimes).

In the weeks that followed, I gave Betsy the correct word for *dick,* and both of us substituted the word *penis* in our work together. She started having some more vivid dreams of her abuse and frequently woke up Miss Mary just to make sure she was dreaming. She continued to visit her aunt and cousins and seemed hypervigilant when the teenage boys were around with her cousins. One day she asked Marlene if she had seen her boyfriend's penis. Marlene said she had not, and it was not appropriate for him to be showing his penis to her. (I must say that Estela and her children were perfect co-therapists and always seemed to have wonderful intuitive responses that were "just right.")

Another child I had worked with had done some great work making penises out of clay that we later dressed up and gave names to. I thought this might be a good intervention for Betsy, and she was initially very invested in making the penises out of brown clay. I remember that she stood one up on the table, squishing it down so that it would stick. Then she picked it up and laid it down on the table. "Penises sleep sometimes, and then they wake up." When I asked her to show me what that looked like, she took the penis that was horizontal and put her hands around the penis and started to move her hands up and down. When she did this, she looked at me almost frightened. "It looks like someone showed you how to move your hands to make the penis wake up." She would not look back at the clay penis and stopped the movement. She looked at me and said, "I'm so gross." Again I responded, "These men are gross to make you touch their penises." She got up and moved away from the table. "I hate him," she said in the softest little voice. "Sounds like you're angry at him." "He's a bad, bad man, and I hate him." "I understand," I said, "and I think you're a little mad too." I went over to the table, and I said, "I wonder how we might show these penises that we're just a little bit mad." She came over, grabbed an empty coke can, and began to squish the clay. "That's one way," I said. Then she took her fist and punched it over and over. This looked like a good cathartic release, and I asked her to put words to her punches. "If your fists could talk, what would they be saying?" She said, "You can't do that to me anymore. You can't do that to me!" She grabbed up the brown clay and threw it in the trash can. "Be gone," she said. I repeated what she said.

After this session, she asked lots of questions about why she had been abused, why men think to do that, why penises are so bad, and on and on. She asked if penises were ever nice. The questions came fast and furious, and I did the best I could to answer them all: "She was abused because she was there, no other reason"; "Men have problems in their thinking that causes them to make bad choices and hurt people"; "Penises were not made to be bad and hurtful"; "Some penises are nice and respectful to others."

She posed yet other questions: "Do I have to do these gross things when I get married?" and "Did you ever see a penis?"

Whew! I gulped. "By the time you are all grown up, after you go to elementary school, high school, and college and you are a grown-up woman, you may meet someone that you grow to love. When people love each other, they use their bodies to show that love to each other. That's called making love. Making love is very, very different from being abused. You will not have to worry about this for a long, long time."

And, finally (gulp, gulp), "When I was a grown-up woman, I met the man that I married and when you marry you show love to each other in lots of ways. So yes, when I married my husband I met a nice penis, and so I have seen one that was nice and did not hurt me or anyone else."

I usually don't answer personal questions. This answer was a huge exception, but in the context of the work that we were doing, I felt it necessary to respond to her. I am happy to report that Betsy understood what I had said. I know that because about a year later she told Estela about our conversation, and Estela was able to add that she, too, had fallen in love with a wonderful man with a nice and gentle penis that never hurt her or anyone else.

The penis work continued for about 2 months. Betsy had a habit of making clay penises or drawing them and then destroying them. Sometimes she cut out pictures of monster-like figures, drew, cut, and pasted big ugly penises with claws, and then shredded the pictures into little pieces. Later, she put a clay penis inside a jail-like box that had a lock and key to open and close the door that had bars on it. She would put the penis in jail and pretend to be a judge by putting a cape on herself. She would declare, "And you and your nasty penis can go to hell, I mean jail, for the rest of your life." I would often repeat what she said, and I noticed that her voice was getting more and more expressive and loud. But there were other times too, when she would appeal to the penis in the jail to answer her questions, "Why did you do that to me, Daddy?" and "Why did you let those other men use me like a rag doll?" She told me once, "He doesn't have

the answers, but I told him he had to think about it until he does."
One day she told me with a chuckle, "He is in permanent time-out!"

Another poignant moment came when she stuck a small female
figurine in the same jail cell with the penis she referred to as her
father. She stood next to the little box, bringing it toward her face
with her hands. "Now I don't have either of you. You're both gone
to me." She would put it down and seem sad for a while. I would
always say to her, "It's not easy to have both your parents gone." She
never responded, but then one day she brought another female figure
into the jail and had her talk to the mother and father figures there.
"Your loss, my gain." I could only assume this was either Miss Mary
or Estela.

Posttraumatic play was evident for many months, but as questions surfaced, the opportunity for psychoeducation arose. In addition, some of the creative, sensory work of making the clay penises
resulted in Betsy verbalizing some of the sexual activities she had
witnessed or experienced. As those memories surfaced, we were able
to trace her thoughts, feelings, and sensations as well as her defensive
mechanism throughout her abuse. She used a form of depersonalization in which she imagined herself a wooden statue that could not be
broken or hurt. "You know those wooden statues you see of cowboys
and Indians and their horses?" I think I knew what she meant, but
she would add, "Those are so hard, they're like cement." One day
she used a shield on her chest and one on her back and asked me to
find pieces of wood she could put on her legs. I had my husband cut
up some pieces of wood that were the right size, and we tied them
around her legs. She stood in place for the longest time and said, "I'm
still here, you just can't see me." She described this invisibility as
something she achieved quickly and easily. It was clear that her defensive strategies had been in place early and had served her well. She
noted that she hardly ever pretended to be wooden anymore because
"I just don't need it anymore."

We also worked on some of Betsy's cognitive distortions such as
the fact that she had caused her dad to become bad, that all penises
would hurt her, and that she would have to subject herself to abuse in
the future. As we did this work, she relaxed more around her cousins'
boyfriends, and her anxiety around men decreased in general. Estela
dated a man occasionally, and this gave Betsy another opportunity

to see that men could be kind and safe. Betsy also developed a warm relationship to a male teacher in her school whom she insisted she had met before but didn't remember where or when.

I cannot be happier to report that a year into our therapy, Estela made a permanent commitment to Betsy and became her adoptive mother. I attended the adoption ceremony at court and later at a restaurant where I joined them for pizza. Betsy had made great progress and now allowed herself to depend on Estela more and more. After our individual therapy and prior to the adoption, we had some parent–child conjoint meetings between Estela and Betsy, some family therapy meetings with Estela, Betsy, and Miss Mary, and some family therapy meetings with Estela, Marlene, and Charlene.

I continued to work with Betsy for another year, although not always on a weekly basis. She had the expected "honeymoon period" with her new family, and then a few challenging behaviors emerged. Her cousins were accepting and provided empathic responses even when they found her strange and annoying. Estela was a pillar of strength and commitment. This child began to experience a normative family life with some regression for a period of time (she wanted to sleep with her mom, she would use baby language, she wanted her mom to comb her hair and put her to bed every night). Estela's instincts were impeccable, and Betsy's comfort and sense of safety and security grew by leaps and bounds. I felt confident that whatever challenge arose, Estela had established a strong foundation and would find the right way to proceed. My confidence in her was only matched by her belief that she had made the right decision to adopt her older sister's only child and give her the life that Laura had never achieved.

CONCLUSION

Chronic sexual abuse can have long-lasting repercussions, although children learn to adopt varied and creative ways to survive. This 9-year-old girl was able to dissociate sufficiently to remove herself from the immediacy of the pain and distress of situations. At the same time, dissociation is by definition a form of compartmentalizing that makes the traumatic experience difficult to integrate into a coherent memory. Without such coherence, fragments of the experience can persist, and processing will be unattainable. It became important for this child to have a therapeutic experience of remembering and managing traumatic experiences. She chose posttraumatic play to reenact her memories, discharge affect, and transform her wooden helplessness into an active and dynamic restoration of power and control. Betsy was unique in her lack of traditional symptoms: She achieved adaptation through invisibility, compliance, and rolling with the punches. She had been on her own from a very young age and was very self-reliant. In a way, she was pseudo-mature, giving a false impression of her strength. Through posttraumatic play, she encountered her emotions and found ways to show them. She posed questions that most children don't even imagine, and she was able to accept the love and affection of family members who met her where she was. They never judged or hurried her; they simply invited her to become family. This case warms my heart.

—— *12* ——

The Terror of Bullying

Maddie C. was 12 years old when I first met her. This chapter involves her experiences in seventh grade. Maddie was referred for therapy by her school counselor, Mrs. D., who felt strongly that Maddie needed to see a therapist due to her depression and lack of interest in school. She was quick to point out that Maddie continued to get decent grades but that she was "skating along," without really trying. According to Mrs. D., Maddie was very smart and could make straight "A's" if she applied herself, but she had changed greatly in the past two school years. Mrs. D. "sensed" that something was terribly wrong but she couldn't guess what that could be. She had established a good relationship with Maddie's parents, who were very invested in their child and were very much "by the book." Mrs. D. stated that Maddie's parents were very concerned about her and thus followed her recommendations for therapy swiftly.

INTAKE INTERVIEW

Mrs. D. was correct about the parents and their concern about their daughter. They, too, had noticed changes in her behavior and asked her numerous times if everything was okay. They described her as a "perfect" child, who gave them little trouble. After her three brothers and sisters were born, she became the perfect big sister, and her parents described a smooth childhood in every way. Maddie's mother had a normal pregnancy, and Maddie was born on time, with no medical concerns. She breastfed well for a few months and her mother transitioned her to bottles without fuss. Mrs. C.'s mother spent the first 2 years with this child and with each of her other grandchildren. This allowed the parents to work without too much interruption, after a brief period of maternity and paternity leaves from their employers. Both Mr. and Mrs. C. were well educated and had met in college. They had graduate degrees and specialized in computer technology. They had very good jobs at separate corporations and enjoyed successful careers that allowed them to take yearly vacations with their four children.

The parents talked about Maddie's weight gain with confusion. They did not understand what was causing her to eat so much and hide food in her room. They had not known what to do about this issue and seemed embarrassed that their daughter was a full 50 pounds overweight, which had caused her pediatrician to label her "grossly obese." Her parents said they had tried many things to help Maddie, but she had become increasingly withdrawn and noncompliant. Mrs. C. said that she was now afraid to talk to her daughter about her weight because she usually broke down in tears and cried inconsolably. Mr. C. said that they had discussed bringing Maddie for therapy for almost a year but had not followed through until Mrs. D. gave them a specific name and phone number. Mrs. D.'s concerns had troubled them and also convinced them that something was bothering Maddie and that she needed professional help. Mrs. D. told Maddie's parents that Maddie was often teased by some of her classmates and that she isolated herself from others, frequently looking sad and despondent. During the intake session, Maddie's parents asked for direction on how to help Maddie with her weight gain. In addition, they wanted help in reopening their lines of communication; they had had a close relationship to their daughter when she was younger and wanted to get back to the comfort they had with her. At this point, Maddie's parents felt that they couldn't reach her and that something was bothering her that she would not share with them.

INDIVIDUAL MEETINGS WITH MADDIE

To say that Maddie appeared sad was an understatement. I immediately understood Mrs. D.'s concerns about this child. She barely made eye contact, she spoke so softly that I could not understand her, and she seemed disinterested in exploring the room. I had asked her parents ahead of time if there was anything that Maddie liked to do, and they commented on her interest in other countries. I had grabbed some *National Geographic* magazines and had a large globe in the office that I displayed more prominently. I also told her that I was from a different country, the way her grandparents and parents— from China—were. As a matter of fact, I told her, both my parents were Ecuadorian. I asked if she had been to China, and she told me she usually went to see her grandparents during summer vacations. I told her that I spoke Spanish and wondered if she spoke Chinese. She said she did and that her grandmother had taught her when she was little.

The first few sessions were painful. Maddie seemed so uncomfortable in her body, and every interaction seemed awkward for her. Her discomfort was such that it made me uncomfortable, and I found myself working harder than I usually did.

Externalization and Containment

Maddie asked if I had Barbie dolls, saying her mother did not let her play with them. I told her I had one Barbie doll and took it out of storage for her. Her play with this doll was unusual: She both undressed her and lowered her fingers around her body and banged her against the desk. She banged her so hard that I had to ask her to slow down, since she was putting marks on the desk. She asked for two more Barbies, and I scrounged through storage to find two more dolls. Once she had the three, she settled into a particular sequence of play that became repetitive and highly structured. Each time she came, she did the following:

> Took out the dolls, undressed them, and threw away the clothes.
> Took the dolls and put them inside a desk.
> Took a bathroom break.
> Scared the three dolls with a two-headed dragon.
> Nurtured a small brown doll and combed her black hair.
> Left the dolls out of sight and left the session.

Each sequence took between 5 and 10 minutes. She looked at the dolls intently. She was very quiet throughout except for putting the dolls inside the desk and pushing the top down briskly. She also had the two-headed dragon roar loudly at the dolls inside the desk. When she nurtured her doll, she held her close and hummed to her.

This play continued for quite a while, perhaps for 10 to 12 sessions. During that time Maddie began to make more eye contact and smiled from time to time. Her smiles were fleeting. When Maddie nurtured the doll, she seemed distant and almost trance-like. After carefully documenting the sequence of her play, I also checked with school and home to see how Maddie was doing in both settings. Parents found her the same, with little change. Mrs. D. said that Maddie's teachers were finding Maddie more distracted, more emotional, and less focused. They were concerned that she might be getting worse.

I was interested to see how her play evolved and became more definitive as her role became more active: There were three dolls who were hidden, and a monster found them and scared them. Separate from that sequence of play, she found it important to nurture a fourth doll as if it were a young baby who needed comfort and protection. Intuitively, based on her behaviors in the therapy office, I began to suspect that something was happening to Maddie with her siblings (three dolls and three siblings and the introduction of a protective parent might have been a wish for her mother to become more involved and more nurturing). I began to make descriptive comments on the play, which she didn't like my doing initially (she looked up with a look of frustration) but later ignored me for the most part. I made open-ended statements such as, "I wonder who the girls are," and "I wonder if the girls are friends to each other or sisters." She did not respond. To my statement "I wonder what the girls are doing inside the desk," she replied: "The girls are inside the desk without their clothes on . . . someone took their clothes off." She also stated calmly, "The two-headed dragon is roaring at those girls." I said, "I'm guessing the girls are afraid when the two-headed dragon comes around and roars." She was mostly unresponsive, but when I commented that she was "holding the baby and singing to her," she looked over at me and stated, "She's not scared, she's brave." I responded, "She's brave in her mommy's arms." "She's brave anyway," she quipped.

One day I asked: "What's it like for those girls when the two-headed dragon comes around?" Finally, she responded, "Those are bad girls; they deserve to suffer." The first few times I repeated what she said. Then I asked "What have these girls done to deserve to suffer?" She held the baby closer to her and said, "They make her life miserable." After this exchange, Maddie became more verbal and also drew some powerful pictures that she tore up before she left the session. The pictures showed three girls hitting and hurting a child in a bathroom. They would force her to take off her clothes, and they would slap her breasts and pinch her, leaving marks on her chest and stomach. They also made her pee in front of them, and they laughed and laughed, saying mean things about how "gross" the girl was on the toilet. This play was compelling, repetitive, and intense. Maddie's affect was constricted, and she often dissociated while looking at the girls in the desk.

I began to express concern for the girls each time they would be undressed inside the desk. "I'm worried about them, I bet no one even knows they're locked up," and "I'm sure those girls hate someone taking off their clothes." I encouraged Maddie to take an empathic stance when thinking about the nude girls in the desk, even though they were mean. "No one deserves to be kept nude and locked up," I offered. "They do! They are very mean!" I kept making empathic comments because I thought that Maddie was beginning to follow my lead. "Mean people are not born mean," I said. "They must be very unhappy people." "No," she would say, "they're just mean. No need to feel sorry for them." I saw an opening and took it, "Who should we feel sorry for?" Maddie replied, "The real girl they do this to . . . " "Oh, my," I said to Maddie, "I hate knowing that there's a real child who's being hurt and we can't help her." "Why can't we help her?" she asked earnestly. "Well . . . because we don't know who she is." "What if I tell you?" Maddie said. I measured my words carefully, "Then we'll try really hard to help her." "But if I tell," Maddie said, using the first person, "they will hurt me even more and show pictures of me peeing to everybody." I came close to her, held her hands in mine, and said gently, "If there are girls hurting you, Maddie, taking off your clothes, pinching you, making you pee in front of them, or taking pictures of you, I will make sure that the abuse stops." I went on to say, "Mean girls are mean because they think no one can stop them. But if they are hurting you, Maddie, we will let the school know, and we will stop them from hurting you again." "You can't stop them," Maddie said, "they are really, really mean and really, really strong." I reassured her that her parents, her teachers, her principals, and I would be much stronger than three mean girls!

Eventually, Maddie disclosed the names of the girls who had been brutalizing her throughout the school year, and the school personnel took her complaints seriously. At first, the school social worker who referred her was incredulous that these events could take place without someone noticing—the principal had also hesitated when first hearing Maddie's allegations. It's important to note that this was one of the earliest cases of bullying documented in the geographic area where I worked, so very few of the current precautionary measures were in place. Awareness of the extent of this type of aggressive activity was not yet well known.

By the time the police interrogated Maddie, she was confident of her parents' support, and her teachers had offered their sincere apologies for failing to protect her. The school personnel suspended the three culprits, and later on, they were expelled and referred for intensive therapy. Maddie spoke clearly about the three classmates who started out by teasing her and later cornered her in the bathroom, where they made her take off her top and pinched her in the breasts and stomach. These girls were relentless in pointing out Maddie's weight gain (highly correlated to the ongoing stress she was under) and told her she smelled. They said they could smell her coming and knew when she wasn't at school because it smelled better.

Their abuse was without precedent in my experience: They called her names, they stole her lunch food and lunch money, they threatened to pull all her clothes off, and they tripped her and stepped on her feet. The floodgates opened as Maddie made clear that she had been living in a chronically traumatic situation. Mr. and Mrs. C. were devastated when I called them into my office and told them what I had discovered and the action I would be taking to notify authorities who could investigate the situation. I told them how difficult it had been for Maddie to speak about her situation and how full of fear she was. I asked for their patience to prepare Maddie to talk with them directly. Maddie was aware that I would be talking to her parents and the police and seemed concerned, but she accepted what I had told her—namely, that she deserved to be safe and secure in her school and that the girls in question needed to be stopped from hurting anyone else. I coached the parents to simply tell Maddie that they had met with me and heard about the terrible situation that was going on at school and that they understood that she felt afraid to tell them what was going on.

The parents and I had discussed their keeping her home from school while I made the report and authorities interviewed school personnel, but the parents felt that it would be better for her not to return to the school where so much abuse had taken place. Maddie felt immense gratitude to her parents for taking her out of the school she dreaded. She was eager to go to another school and start anew in a safer setting. I continued to see Maddie during her transition to her new school.

MADDIE'S PLAY CHANGES: RELEASE OF ENERGY AND ACTIVATION OF RESOURCES

Maddie used a magic wand and gave herself a wizard name, Chelsea. As Chelsea, she cast spells and turned the bad children into good ones and the good ones into bad ones. When the good children turned bad, they would do hateful things to their friends. They would hide their food, cut their hair, and push them down and step on them. Meanwhile the bad girls turned good, begged the wizard to help and keep the children safe. The play became very frenetic, and it was hard to know what was going on. Maddie's speech became pressured, her movements became jerky, and at times, she stopped and stared at the dolls in front of her, becoming less present and less available in the room. The play intensified in the following weeks and she was clearly distressed, as the play seemed to evolve without the rigid control and structure she had exercised earlier in the treatment. I interpreted this as a good sign since she seemed to release energy when she challenged the constriction of her affect and movements in the past. My guess was that not being at the school and gaining distance from massive stress, she was now able to externalize some of her abuse. In addition, she was feeling empowered by her parents' support. They reported that she was more outgoing with them and was seeking them out for comfort. Mr. and Mrs. C. were alarmed at the extent of the abuse that Maddie disclosed and told her they would call the police with new information. The police were highly supportive of the parents. One of the officers developed a special relationship to Maddie, frequently checking in on her to see how she was doing in her new school.

Luckily, for Maddie, the girls readily admitted to their brash cruelty, and so Maddie did not need to prove that the abuse had occurred. Her parents were satisfied with the expulsion and did not want their daughter to be exposed to additional confrontations; they also expressed satisfaction with the school's new policies and procedures. The principal, teacher, and social worker had visited Maddie to thank her for being brave enough to speak out about what was going on. They told her that because of her bravery, other children would now be safe and the mean girls would get the help they needed to stop hurting others.

Maddie also received a letter from each of the three girls who had tortured her. They apologized for a series of cruel, sadistic behaviors and told Maddie she had done nothing to elicit this hatred from them. Maddie read the letter and asked me to keep it for her. She said she didn't want it in her house because it had been written by her tormentors, but she might want to reread it sometime in the future.

During her posttraumatic play, as described earlier, Maddie found her voice. In the role of Chelsea, the wizard, she punished the mean girls without mercy. She had one of the "mean girls" do to them all the things they had done to her, and then some. She sometimes laughed when the victim doll cried or protested. She sometimes threw the good girl against the wall, telling her to "toughen up!" and asking her "why" she had been such a doormat. In addition, during a few sessions she had Chelsea place a different type of spell on the victim child (there was only one victim at a time). The new spell made the victim child grow "Infinite Powers of the Brain, the Heart, and the Muscle." This buffered-up victim could blow her victimizers away, could cause them to explode into a million pieces by holding her breath, and could tie them up and send them to an island where they could only survive by their wits. ("I will leave them some little wits so they can grow them," she whispered in my ear.)

AGE-APPROPRIATE RESOLUTION AND CLOSURE

Maddie was ultimately able to express her fears and worries, her hopes and wishes, and likewise reveal all the negative thinking that seemed to contribute to her being overweight. "You are ugly and smelly," she would tell the victim, and "You'll never amount to anything," and "No one cares about you or even notices that you've got scars all over your ugly body." She was teased consistently for being overweight, for being dumb, and sometimes for being Chinese and a "foreigner." The victimizers had managed to tear her down and strip her of her pride and her sense of self-esteem. The fact that she could not turn to her parents for help had left her isolated and vulnerable to the daily humiliations she endured.

As she played, she became emotionally present; she verbalized and documented an array of abuses, using play to rectify and redirect her aggression. She punished the mean girls to her heart's content, and as she did so she allowed a great deal of emotional intensity to fill the room. Little by little, she was transforming her sense of herself as a victim to a more powerful girl, capable of self-protection. She was able to respond to her abusers, yelling firmly that she did not smell, that she was not stupid—and one last one that I liked in particular: "I may be a little fat, but I can lose the weight; you can't lose the meanness!!" She had started naturally to talk about how parents could help the victim child, and I suggested that we bring in her parents so that she could say as much or as little to them about the abuse she had endured. At this juncture, there was a coherent narrative, her memories had been processed, she had expressed her fears and worries, and she had reclaimed her sense of goodness and fairness.

Maddie asked if she would have to tell her parents everything that happened to her, and I told her she just had to say as much or as little as she wanted to in order to have her parents understand what she had endured and be available to her anytime she needed. Maddie agreed, and we spent two sessions making notes on note cards about what she wanted to share. Even this process of selecting what to tell her parents included empathic and thoughtful selections that would protect her parents from knowing too much. It's important to note that during her posttraumatic play, Chelsea the Wizard cast a spell of blindness on the parents and teachers and then reversed it. Maddie had managed to show that even though she was proud that her parents had moved her out of the school where she was abused, she was angry at them for not knowing that she was in trouble. The bullying girls had threatened Maddie's siblings with harm if Maddie told her parents about the abuse. One of Maddie's sisters was in a lower grade, and Maddie was petrified that they would bring her into the abuse. This ability and willingness to keep her sister safe helped renew her self-esteem.

JOINT SESSIONS

As mentioned earlier, Maddie seemed ready to talk to her parents about the details of what she had endured. Mr. and Mrs. C. had a general understanding of the abuse, but it seemed relevant for them to hear a little more so that Maddie could fully use them as a resource going forward. In addition, I believe it was important for Maddie to receive comfort and reassurance from her parents, and the hope going into these sessions was that this reassurance would occur.

For her part, Mrs. C. had to overcome the debilitating sense of guilt she had over not knowing what was going on. She had berated herself for not recognizing the physical signs of abuse. She had not even considered the possibility that her child was being abused, instead focusing on the child's obesity. When Maddie covered up the scars on her body, her mother simply thought that she was covering up because she was self-conscious about her body and being overweight. Mrs. C. was anxious about these meetings, and both Mrs. C.'s own therapist and I helped prepare her to focus on her child's needs during these meetings. Mr. C. felt eager to listen and was happy that his daughter was communicating with them more clearly.

The sessions were challenging, poignant, and successful. Maddie stayed in control of what happened in the session, and her parents agreed to whatever she wanted. Sometimes Maddie would simply use her note cards and give them "facts," and other times, she would tell stories with the dolls in the room. She never showed them all of her stories, and she remained much more subdued as she talked to her parents. But she was able to talk to them directly about how angry she was that they had failed to recognize that she needed help. Her parents apologized in a genuine and trustworthy way. It was clear they were putting Maddie's needs far ahead of their own. Maddie soaked up their empathic responses. There was very little physical contact between them, but sometimes they held hands as they left the office. Maddie talked to her parents about how she would "signal" that there was a problem at school even if she couldn't talk to them in detail. They came up with the use of a red card that she would give to her parents if she was in distress. When her parents asked what to do if she shut herself down again, Maddie told them to ask her to write things down and she would deliver letters and notes to them if something was scaring or hurting her.

CONCLUSION

Maddie's symptoms were moderate, but she did not escape the watchful eye of the school social worker who developed concern about sudden changes in Maddie's school behaviors. Her intuition told her that something had gone awry in Maddie's life, and so she called the parents and gave them a referral for therapy.

Maddie was able to utilize posttraumatic play to pull herself out of a position of helplessness and develop mastery and personal control over an overwhelmingly difficult and painful situation. Her play was simultaneously symbolic and literal, and it became more and more dynamic over time. Maddie was able to infuse the repetitive play with differences and clearly used it both to acknowledge the pervasive helplessness and to dole out justice for those who had so severely hurt her over months. Maddie did in play what she could not do in real life, and once the play provided release and relief, her family was invited to learn more about her experiences and how they could help her.

The joint sessions were effective and powerful for all family members. They enabled Maddie to regain confidence, believe in herself and the goodness of others, and accept the warmth of her family, including her siblings. The acute crisis was over, and Maddie had transitioned to a less vulnerable and more self-efficient young child. Because several PTSD symptoms persisted for a period of time, Maddie participated in group therapy with other abused children. Meeting and interacting with other child victims helped her feel less stigmatized and more confident that she had not been singled out for any particular personal traits other than her vulnerability and "softness," which she considered good traits.

— *13* —

"I Will Come Out by Myself"

Sharelle was chronologically 4 years of age and developmentally closer to 2 when I first met her. She was in her second foster care placement and had been removed from her birth parents at age 2 due to severe neglect. Her current foster mother, Mrs. S., had cared for Sharelle for 10 months. Her first foster parent became ill and requested the child's removal. Mrs. S. had recently telephoned the DFS in a panic. She stated that she needed help because Sharelle did not appear to be making any progress and was still unresponsive, cried a lot, and difficult to comfort. Mrs. S. felt that Sharelle was not "connecting" with her, and she found herself feeling despair. Mrs. S. began to feel that Sharelle simply did not like her, and she told the social worker that perhaps it would be best to place the child in yet another home. The social worker, correctly, was loath to move the child again and instead referred Mrs. S. and Sharelle to therapy to determine whether Sharelle could be helped to change some of her behaviors, specifically "attachment issues with her foster mother," and so prevent another placement.

INTAKE SESSION

I met with Mrs. S. and found her to be forthcoming and invested in Sharelle. Mrs. S. was a foster parent who was eager to adopt a young child that she "could call her own." Mrs. S. told a heartbreaking story of trying to adopt another young child in her care and having a relative show up shortly before the adoption hearing. She said that she had never felt this kind of pain before but that in the long run, she had understood that the joy of parenting the child trumped the painful feelings she could experience if things did not work out. She described parenting this first foster child as "sheer heaven." As she talked, she articulated her high expectations and her desire for unconditional love from a child. It was not surprising then to hear Mrs. S. talk about her deep disappointment about Sharelle's lack of affection, her typical style of withdrawing, and her ongoing fear and anxiety around the house. "By now," she stated with alarm in her voice, "she should be turning to me more and more. God knows I've done everything I could to make her feel safe and comfortable, but no matter what I do, she doesn't change." She went on to say that her biggest concern was that Sharelle never sought her out, never asked her for help, never seemed to need her. As she said this, she cried. It was clear to me that Mrs. S. had lots of love that she wanted to give and was definitely eager to find "the right fit." Our conversation about attachment and early trauma was intellectual, and I noticed this mother's detached understanding.

Mrs. S. told me about all the courses she had taken and all the articles she had read. It was clear she had gone above and beyond an expectable level of education on the topic of attachment. Unfortunately, somewhere along the line her expectations became inflated, and she believed that the child was young enough to be receptive to her nurturing behaviors, as long as she was consistent and empathic. Mrs. S. took out her phone to show me a tape of her reading to Sharelle before bedtime, and Sharelle wanting to stay under her covers, refusing to cuddle, and looking away as Mrs. S. read the book. She showed me this as a "glaring example" of Sharelle's issues with her. It was clear to me that she was interpreting Sharelle's behavior as a rejection and personalizing Sharelle's attempts to protect herself with an unfamiliar person and establish trust and safety.

Before she left, I asked Mrs. S. about her current feelings about the child. "I fell in love with her the moment I saw her," she said emphatically, and then added, "I still love her, but I want her to love me back. I feel so lonely and pushed away." Of course, I told Mrs. S. that she was doing the right thing in not giving up, that her consistency could pay off, and that I would do what I could to help. We set up the appointment schedule with Sharelle, and I asked the social worker to send me whatever paper trail existed on Sharelle and what had initially brought her into foster care. I had asked Mrs. S. what she knew about Sharelle's early development, and she told me that she didn't know the details but knew that Sharelle had been neglected, malnourished, and unsupervised. (I later found the details more extensive and disturbing.)

BEGINNING THERAPY

Sharelle did not hold Mrs. S.'s hand as they went into the waiting room and sat down next to her with her thumb in her mouth. She looked around the room with controlled vigilance. I noticed she was quite still. I asked her if she wanted to come into the office alone (with me) or with Mrs. S., and she just walked into the room I had emerged from. I followed her quickly but not before I noticed the look of hurt in Mrs. S.'s eyes as Sharelle left without a word or a glance in her direction.

I showed her around, told her who I was, and asked her if she knew why she was coming to see me. She shook her head no. Mrs. S. had told me that Sharelle was very quiet and used few words. I said a few things: my name, that I worked with children, and that I was there to get to know her a little and see how she was feeling about living with Mrs. S. She ignored me.

I took her around the room by the hand, which she offered freely, and I pointed out several age-appropriate games or toys in the room, since she had expressed atypical disinterest in the toys. She did not seem eager but did go over to the easel and wanted to use the paints to make a picture. She made circles of different colors and made sure the paints did not touch, which I thought showed a great deal of control for a child of 4 years and a few months. She never mixed the paints, stood back quietly, used all the colors available to her, and then stopped.

I had an office that was divided into two rooms separated by an opening where a door had been. The first office had a couch and chairs, and the second room was the play therapy office. After she painted, she came out into the first room and climbed into the couch and stared out without a word. She sucked her thumb and seemed perfectly content. I took a seat next to her and did parallel play, also staring out in a relaxed fashion. She never turned her head to look at me, but she did give me some sideways glances. We spent about 15 minutes this way in our first session, and then it was time to leave. I told her it was time and that I would see her the following week. She walked out the door, past Mrs. S., and left the waiting room. Mrs. S. followed behind her, asking her to take her hand. I looked down the hall to see the child reluctantly taking Mrs. S.'s hand.

EARLY SESSIONS

In our subsequent sessions, Sharelle moved and explored slowly. She was extremely hypervigilant and noticed every single sound in the room. My office had an unusual heating/cooling system overhead that went on loudly and did not appear to have a consistent time-frame for going on and off. Sharelle also looked up when she heard footsteps, in spite of the fact that a sound machine was outside the door to muffle sounds and decrease interruptions. I also shared a wall with another therapist, and every now and then she heard voices and seemed to listen for a while with attention, and then she would retreat into thumbsucking.

Sharelle developed a routine in the first six sessions in which she would come into the play therapy office first, then stand and look around, as if taking stock of the toys in the room. Sometimes I wondered if she was taking in the consistency of the toys or noticing if things were out of place. A few times I commented that something was out of place and put it in its place. Once I noticed that she put a bear in its bin with other bears. She spoke few words, and her eyes and body remained consistently still and fixed.

During most sessions, she would sit on the couch for about half the time and look out as I sat next to her. On or about the seventh meeting, I brought out some bubbles and blew them into the air. I directed them toward her, and they floated by. She followed them with her eyes. I blew lots of little bubbles that went everywhere. I also tried to form larger bubbles and would blow a large circle into the room. I got up a few times and blew the big bubble around. She was watching cautiously. Another time I got up and started trying to catch the bubbles. I could have sworn I heard the slightest hint of a very quiet giggle once, but if I did, it was short-lived. Next, I blew some bubbles so that they would land near me. I tried to catch the bubbles on my hand, and they would pop. Finally, I blew a bubble so that it would land on her knee. It sat there for a while. I commented that the bubble had not popped and was staying on her knee a long time. Finally, it popped, and when it did, she took her little finger and touched the wet place where the bubble had been. I was encouraged by these very small signs of physical movement and the energy it implied.

I continued sitting with her and blowing bubbles for a few more sessions, and she continued painting when she first came in and after she perused the room. We had developed a comfortable and predictable environment, and she knew that I would not bother her asking questions and expecting her to respond verbally. Instead, I assessed her physical movement, her breathing, her gaze, the smallest of changes in her behavior. For example, I noticed that she took a very pronounced step when crossing the strip of steel that separated one room from another. This barrier seemed relevant to her, and she always stopped before crossing it.

By about the fourth month, Sharelle seemed more relaxed, carried herself with less tension, and seemed to breathe more easily. She and I had a routine, a way of being together that placed few demands on her. She liked to come into the room, look around, move a few things, paint (sometimes), and then sit in the corner of the room. Sometimes she sat for 15 to 20 minutes, other times for just a couple of minutes, but sitting down seemed important to her whether she was still or active. Sharelle was tolerating the new therapy environment well.

Mrs. S. told me that on Thursdays, the day of our therapy session, Sharelle looked for her jacket and sat by the door, signaling that she knew it was time to go to the sessions. Mrs. S. said that a "pretty spectacular change" had happened at home, but she was trying not to get too excited about it because she was afraid it could be taken away from her as quickly as it came. She described the change, and it seemed important to me as well. I had asked Mrs. S. to incorporate no more and no less than 10 minutes of rocking with her each night. Mrs. S. initially said that Sharelle did not tolerate being held at all, and I encouraged her to get on the chair, allow Sharelle to hold her own stuffed animal, and tell Sharelle that her baby bear needed to be rocked. Sharelle had picked out the same baby bear each time for rocking, and because Mrs. S. did this before bedtime, Sharelle was getting the bear without being instructed to do so. I had also asked Mrs. S. to put on a timer for 10 minutes. By the end of the first month of this daily behavior, Sharelle asked for "more," and the alarm was set for 15, then 20 minutes. I thought this was a great improvement, and Mrs. S. was ecstatic when Sharelle asked for more time on her lap.

It was remarkable to me that Mrs. S. could not fully enjoy this recent change in Sharelle's receptivity to closeness because she was afraid it could suddenly stop. This inability to live in the present and persistent expectation of failure troubled me, and I told her that someone in our office could be available to see her at the same time that Sharelle came in to see me. At first, Mrs. S. seemed surprised by my suggestion of therapy for her, upon which I offered her my rationale: An incredible desire to give her heart to Sharelle, coupled with panic that her heart could be broken, often immobilized her and kept her from making a full investment and feeling hopeful. She agreed, and when she began to share her predictable history of loss (of a primary attachment figure) early on in her life, I pointed out that her history was important to revisit so that she could achieve some kind of closure and move on. Her last words to me in that session were, "I know I wouldn't be so afraid if it wasn't for the fact I was left alone so early in my life." I remember telling her that she and Sharelle had something in common, and now she would have the opportunity to give to this little girl what she had sorely missed. She agreed to therapy, and the parallel treatment was invaluable.

BEGINNING POSTTRAUMATIC PLAY: EXTERNALIZATION AND CONTAINMENT

At about the fifth month of meeting with Sharelle, a new behavior emerged. When she approached the floor barrier between rooms, she stopped as always, but now she sat down with her body in one room and her legs in the other. She held her stuffed bear and sucked her thumb. This occurred when we were walking to my office to sit on the couch after her exploratory play in the play therapy office and after she had touched and moved the toys, especially attentive to misplaced objects. She liked sitting on the couch and instructed me to "go" in the big room to wait for her (by putting out her index finger). I followed her directives and sat there watching her little legs until she chose to stand and join me on the couch.

This routine continued with her showing me her toes, feet and ankles, legs, and eventually one or two hands prior to standing up. She also made "hush" sounds from the other side of the wall. "I hear a hushing sound," I would say, and she would not respond. As time went by, I recognized that silence was relevant in this play, especially her ability to break the silence with noises. At first she would throw something against the wall with a small thud. Eventually, she used a bigger thud. I would simply state that I heard a big thud and a little thud.

When we sat on the couch, we participated in a number of games. We started by popping bubbles with our hands, then with our feet, next with our heads, and so on. She had never smiled or laughed while doing this and her body was quite stiff, but she followed my lead and watched me carefully. Other times we sat together and read a book while listening to music, or we played with colorful cardboard boxes, stacking one on top of the other.

Two important things happened quite serendipitously in this early phase of her posttraumatic play: (1) Sharelle began to make noises on her own, by making a tall tower of cardboard boxes and then knocking them down first with a punch and later with a brisk kick; and (2) after building towers and knocking them over, Sharelle used the boxes to construct a tall square and she sat in the center of it. She asked me to sit on the side of the square so that I could not see her. These behaviors turned out to be relevant to her specific traumas and signaled her earliest attempts to externalize some of the memories that had been kept at bay.

When Sharelle first saw the differently colored cardboard boxes, she ignored them. At this juncture in treatment, she had begun to explore some of the toys in the office, and in one particular session, she took out one of the boxes and set it on the middle of the floor. She laid it down and stood it up several times before she went to get a second, third, and fourth cardboard box. She was small enough that six boxes were about her size, and she seemed to enjoy constructing this tower and standing next to it with her arms by her side, staring forward. During another session a few weeks later, she took her hand, made a little fist, and knocked the cardboard box at the top, then the next, and so forth until she had punched all the boxes. Some of the boxes flew back and some sideways; this was the first time I saw her smile. A few sessions later, she kicked the box with her leg, and when the boxes flew every which way, she giggled. Of course, I giggled with her and said, "Your leg kicked the boxes, and they flew all over the place. He, he, that's funny." She quickly made the tower and kicked it again, this time with definitive laughter coming from her belly. This was one of the best sounds ever, so very uninhibited and genuine. She repeated this kicking motion over and over, always ending with a laugh that we shared. It was clear to me that Sharelle was enjoying the act of creating noise and safe unpredictability, constructing and reconstructing, and sharing a relational moment of laughter.

This behavior gave way to her building a small square on the floor that she would step in and out of. Yet again, when she stepped in, she would stand with her arms to one side, except that now she would look at me and fill her cheeks with air. Then she would spit wind, making another powerful noise that filled the room. Again, she laughed and I laughed with her. Something in Sharelle was being released, and she seemed to be exploring the boundaries of her safety.

Sometimes she sat on the edge of the box, and she would look out. She found a little wooden toy I have of a cat sitting on a ledge fishing (with a fishing rod). She brought that over from its place on the shelf and sat it next to her. Then she positioned her body so that it looked like she was fishing too. More laughter ensued as Sharelle and her little friend sat on the box. She then motioned for me to come over, and I knew it was an important invitation that I wanted to accept. So I sat on the cardboard box as best I could for a few seconds before she stood up and turned around to look at me. She laughed when she saw me crouched down on the box, and then she ran onto the couch after grabbing a book and asked me to come sit with her. I complied, of course.

The walls of the square got higher and higher as Sharelle began to play a game that seemed important to her.

RELEASE OF ENERGY AND ACTIVATION OF RESOURCES

Once the walls were high around her, Sharelle always asked me to sit next to her so that I couldn't see her. She would say "Hello" and I would respond, "Hello, I'm sitting here next to you." Sometimes she would say, "Sssshhhhhh, I'm sleeping," and I would repeat what she said, "Okay, I'm sleeping too." I noticed a few times that she stood up on her tippy toes to look out and make sure I was sleeping. About four or five sessions of this precise play occurred, and then Sharelle said, "I want water." I said, "sure, sounds like you're thirsty, I'll bring you water." And I would go pour her a little water in a small plastic cup and bring to her. She would drink it all up and say, "Ahhhhh, good." She later asked for a snack, so after checking with Mrs. S., she sent special snacks with Sharelle, and we would set them aside until she was ready to incorporate them into her dramatic play. "I need a snack," she would say, and I would bring her a little cup filled with her snack. She began to crunch loudly, which I commented on, and after that, I began to count how many bites she took (that I could hear). She seemed to enjoy this interaction with me, and eventually, her little hand came out of the opening and she would offer me a snack, stating "Only three bites." So I would take three bites and finish the pretzel.

The most profound interactions occurred when Sharelle, sitting in her little box talking with me or asking for things, would say, "Do you know I'm still here?" "You want to make sure I know you're still inside the box. Yes, I know you're there." "Are YOU still there?" "Yes, Sharelle, I'm still here, waiting to know what you would like." One day she said, "I want to hold your fingers." I bent over, because she didn't want me hovering over the box, and I offered my hand. She took two fingers and squeezed them, holding on for what seemed like a long time.

Finally, in this play, she moved over some of the cardboard boxes in the front, and she situated this little container in front of the couch. Now she asked me to read her a book while I sat next to the opening of the box, while she held my fingers. We read about ten books in this fashion.

She then removed the bottom square in her square construction so that the opening was complete in the front. She asked me to sit on the right side of the box. "Can you see my legs?" she would say, as she scooted up in the box, putting her legs in and out. "Yes, I can see your legs," I would say. She would ask, "Are you real or pretend?" "I am real," I would say, "and I can see your legs." Then she hunched over so that her legs reached to her toes. "What do you see now?" "I see your legs and your hands," I responded. After doing this for approximately seven sessions, she stated in the firmest voice I had ever heard from her, "Well, come get me out of here!" I acted quickly and commented on her strong voice. "I'm coming, I'm coming, I hear you." I found her bent over, leaning over herself, hands over toes. I realized she wanted me to pick her up. "I wonder how I will get you out," I asked. "Maybe I'll pick you up." She reached her arms up to me, and I picked her up, bringing her to the couch. She put her arms around my neck, and I patted her back. "You wanted me to get you out of there, and I did." "Yeah," she mumbled and then fell asleep for about 20 minutes. I found myself trying to revisit the play sequences and then stopped myself and simply stayed present, patting her back and humming. When it was time to go, I woke her up gently, and she rubbed her eyes and woke up. I gave her a drink of water and held her hand as we walked out to her foster mother. Without speaking a word, she reached her arms up to Mrs. S. who picked her up. She folded into her arms, looking small and fatigued. "Look at how she's turning to you for warmth and comfort," I said to Mrs. S., and she beamed. She walked out with Sharelle in her arms.

AGE-APPROPRIATE RESOLUTION AND CLOSURE

Sharelle's formal posttraumatic play lasted 7 months, although she exhibited other forms of posttraumatic play in later years, as she became more mature and she made cognitive reassessments of her early experiences.

Toward the end of this second phase of posttraumatic play, I suggested to Mrs. S. that she should buy a little tent for Sharelle and that she should go into the tent with her to play. Mrs. S. made a second purchase of a small tea set and began to have tea parties with Sharelle in the tent. Mrs. S. confided that Sharelle took her by the hand to go into the tent and followed mother's lead when it was time to come out. They had placed a number of Sharelle's favorite books in the tent and usually spent about one full hour prior to Sharelle's bedtime. Mrs. S. was now fully convinced that her decision to adopt Sharelle was the right one, and she no longer doubted that she could be a fine mother to this little girl. In addition, Sharelle had become much more responsive to her and Mrs. S. delighted in this fact.

In our therapy sessions, Sharelle had changed from a very rigid, vigilant, physically constricted, and motionless little girl to a youngster who behaved closer to what was expectable in a child almost 5. She became more curious and more outgoing, and her vocabulary (and willingness to speak) grew.

The play with the box continued into the final phase of post-traumatic play where it became less consistent, less sequential, and more fluid. There were times when she would not build a structure at all, and foregoing the prior sequence, she would ask to play with the dollhouse, the paints, or something else. Other times, when she constructed her structure with boxes, she took all her necessities into the small container, filling it with water, snacks, and a little stuffed bear that she often carried with her and consistently brought to therapy from her house. She called this little Bear "Monique" and told me lots of elaborate stories about her. One such story was so interesting that I chronicled it verbatim in my notes after the session:

> Monique likes the park, but one day a bad man took her hand and took her hard to the basement. She fell down the stairs. Her legs had blood on them, and the puppy licked the blood and got wings and flew away. Then the spiders got inside her ears, and they made strings and mosquitoes bit her ears. Monique got scaredy. She climbed and the room got no windows, dark. Monique sang songs in her head. She heard birdies sing. She made the letter "o" on the floor and the number "3." Sometimes the bad man would find Monique and spank her. Monique's puppy licked her a lot. Monique's mommy told her "Shhhhhh, stay quiet." Monique's mommy didn't help her or take her out. My mommy does. My mommy takes me out to the park, she swings me. She brings snacks for me. Monique is hungry. Let's make food for Monique.

During this last phase of posttraumatic play, Sharelle began to use play more symbolically, and it was evident that Monique was recounting Sharelle's traumatic experiences and Sharelle had become the (pretend) caretaker to her little scared and injured bear. This play was quite important in that, as she provided good care to Monique, she was also providing care to herself, which is an important component of healing. It was also clear to me that Sharelle had now incorporated Mrs. S. as a capable resource for herself, and she happily announced to me that she now had a "forever mom." Mrs. S. handed me the invitation to come to her "adoption hearing and party," and I happily attended. Sharelle's joy could not be contained. She literally jumped up and down with her arms flapping in the air (a difference from the jumping she had done in my office).

Prior to the adoption, however, I felt it would be important for Mrs. S. to perform the function of "unconditional witness" to some of Sharelle's posttraumatic play. I asked Sharelle if it would be alright with her if we invited Mrs. S. to come share some drinks and snacks with her while she sat in her little space. "Yes, yes!" she screamed and went out to the waiting room to ask her mother to come in. I told Sharelle that we would have to wait until the next session, and she seemed disappointed.

I simply asked Mrs. S. to follow her daughter's lead. I wasn't sure exactly what would happen, but I wanted Sharelle to set the pace and lead the way. I had three empty cups with a water bottle, plus some pretzels, on the table. I also took out the cardboard boxes in advance. Sharelle went to work, making the frame and then building it up. She left the front of the box open and then asked her mother to sit on one side and me on the other. True to form, she put her legs out of the box, leaned her body over so that her hands reached the toes, and asked her mom to pick her up. She did this about six times and then asked her mother to come into the house with her to have a snack. I was not invited but was anointed the "waitress" who brought the food and snacks to them. In order for her mother to fit in the structure, they spread out the walls so that it gave a very different feeling than a small container would but continued to offer the semblance of a physical boundary. Mother and daughter happily had their snack. Then Sharelle asked to restore the smaller shape and putting out her legs asked her mom, "Can you see me?" Mrs. S. said, "Yes, I can see you!" "Well, come get me out of here then!" and Mrs. S. got up quickly to hold Sharelle in her arms. Sharelle asked Mom to carry her all the way to the car and Mom agreed.

The reader may find it interesting to note that when I obtained paperwork for this child, there was police documentation that Sharelle had been placed in a closet by her parents and kept there for days at a time without food or water. When she was found in the closet, the officer noted that she did not cry or seem distressed; she just looked around with wide eyes, compliant and receptive. From this description, it appears that she had learned to stay quiet because when someone did come to find her in the closet, physical abuse occurred.

CONCLUSION

Sharelle had experienced cruel and unusual maltreatment as a toddler. She had been unable to verbalize the events that remained vivid in her mind, but she was remarkably adept at utilizing posttraumatic play to re-create the environment of her unique form of abuse: being placed in a closet for days at a time. I only learned about the specifics of her abuse toward the end of therapy; knowing the details made the context of her posttraumatic play vivid and more remarkable. Sharelle found a way to develop enough trust to reach out to me and to her adoptive mother for nurturance and for safety. Her posttraumatic play provided powerful, gradual exposure that she initiated with little prompting. I believe the gentle therapy environment that did not promote a particular agenda but allowed the child time to come forward created an environment conducive to the emergence of posttraumatic play, which included dramatic and symbolic play. There were ample attachment opportunities with both me as her clinician and her eventual adoptive parent.

Other therapy services were provided to this family throughout the child's development, whenever Mrs. S. and Sharelle herself requested them. Over the years we worked on issues such as social skills, impulsivity, loss, anxiety about sexuality, and generalized anxiety in new situations. During her teenage years, Sharelle was especially eager to locate her birth parents, something Mrs. S. found distressing. When Sharelle turned 18, she did indeed obtain more information about her parents, but she opted to forego contact with them.

— 14 —

Conjoint Narrative Sharing

Allyson and her mother, Stephanie, are of Central American descent. Stephanie came with her parents to the United States nearly 10 years earlier when she was 16. Stephanie's mother returned to her country to care for her mother, and Stephanie became the primary caretaker for her four younger siblings. Her father, Carlos, was a good man and a very hard worker. He had three jobs and was barely ever home. Stephanie grew up fast, and she was eager to leave the home and be independent. When her mother returned, she was unable to influence Stephanie to stay at home. Stephanie was 21 when she moved out and used some of her father's contacts to secure a job doing construction work. Her father had taken all the children to work from time to time, and Stephanie had learned some basic skills from him about sheetrocking. She took the first job offered to her and from that point on established her independence. Before long she had a boyfriend, and 6 months into the relationship, she got pregnant with Allyson. Her boyfriend was not interested in having a child and took a job in a nearby state. Stephanie never saw him again.

Stephanie prioritized her daughter's education, wanting her to be more prepared than she had been. She was able to get Allyson into a preschool setting, who thrived in this caring educational environment and was fully bilingual in no time. Her teachers were very

This chapter is adapted from Gil (2015b). Copyright © 2015 The Guilford Press. Adapted by permission.

positive about Allyson's happy and receptive demeanor and felt that her mother was an "amazing young parent." When one of her teachers called me to make a referral for Allyson, her concern was evident, noting that Allyson had changed in almost every way. Allyson did not seem happy, she had become withdrawn and anxious, and she cried throughout the day. This new behavior, and Allyson's inability to acknowledge any specific incident that was causing these concerning behaviors, caused the teacher to call for help.

INTAKE SESSION

I could tell from talking to Stephanie on the phone that something had occurred recently that she was struggling with. Her voice was shaky and she cried on the phone. All she could mutter was that "something horrible, unthinkable" had occurred, and she wanted to get help for her "poor little girl." Of course, initially I thought something had happened to Allyson that had caused her behavioral problems, but it turned out that it was the mother who had sustained the traumatic experience. She had been raped, and the child had witnessed the event, a secondary victim.

Stephanie was distraught, and so I asked her to come to the intake by herself so that we could talk freely. She said she would ask her cousin to take care of her daughter but ended up bringing Allyson to the session, noting that her cousin had canceled. Stephanie added that it was just as well because her daughter was having a very difficult time being separated from her mother for any length of time.

I scheduled Stephanie's return at a time when she could talk freely. At this initial session, then, I instead showed Allyson around the play therapy office, telling her that the next time she came she would have more time to look around and decide what she wanted to play with. Allyson was lively, smiled, and wide-eyed as she looked around the office. Her play quickly turned into posttraumatic play in which she externalized the event that loomed heavy in her mind and that allowed her to release some of her pent-up emotions. This play is chronicled elsewhere (Gil, 2015b). The following details how crucial it was to have a parallel therapeutic process with mother and child, and to bring them together for parent–child family sessions.

INDIVIDUAL WORK WITH MOTHER

It became immediately evident that Stephanie was in acute distress. She hardly seemed able to control her emotions, and she sobbed throughout our early sessions. From the outset, it was evident that she required crisis intervention as well as therapy, and it would be necessary to involve whomever she considered part of her support system. Unfortunately, I quickly discovered that her family was unaware of the rape and thus would not be immediately available to her. She had established a good relationship with a victim advocate who had helped her throughout the medical exam as well as the police investigation and the court trial. Stephanie's willingness to speak to the police in candid fashion and her decision to testify in court allowed for a speedy and full investigation with a successful criminal prosecution.

Stephanie was returning to work slowly but only when her mother was able to take care of her daughter. Stephanie seemed to trust her mother, but there was also a distance in her voice when she spoke of her. She confided in me that she still harbored anger at her mother for leaving her to take care of her younger siblings all by herself. She spoke of her father with greater warmth, but early on she asserted that she would never want either of them to know about what had happened to her. When I asked her why, she answered that they would blame her and would look at her differently. I did not challenge this fear until later in the treatment. Here at the start I only told her that I completely understood her desire to protect her parents from this information.

I told Stephanie that she could say whatever was comfortable for her to say about the rape. I knew she had discussed it in great detail with the police, and I gave her the option of choosing whatever she felt was important for me to know. She described a grueling scene that filled me with fear and anger. She seemed conflicted when she noted that she had allowed a man into her apartment at night. "I don't know what I was thinking," she said, "I don't know how I could have been so stupid." When I suggested that she was being too hard on herself, she energetically emphasized that it was unequivocally wrong for her to have put her child at risk in this way. The man who raped her was brutal and cruel with her, and the rape had lasted approximately three hours, with some brief periods of respite in which he hit her in the stomach and kicked her in the legs and pelvic area.

Throughout this initial disclosure, Stephanie did not mention Allyson. However, at subsequent sessions it became clear that Allyson had seen her mother being raped and beaten, although Stephanie was not able to state unequivocally how much her daughter had witnessed since she was in and out of conscious awareness. She had suffered a skull fracture, concussion, several broken ribs, fractured pelvis, and injuries to her back. When she described the extent of her injuries, it became painfully clear that she had survived a forceful attack by a sick individual. Her resolve to identify him and put him in jail reflected Stephanie's resilient and spirited nature.

From this point on, I opted to work individually with Stephanie and with her daughter. Both were bilingual and required a bilingual therapist to be able to shift with them from Spanish to English easily. Stephanie described having several sessions with an interpreter and how stressful that had been for her. She noted (which is my own personal experience as well) that when she was under acute stress, she spoke most easily in her first language and found translating difficult and tiring. My decision to work with her directly was based on two factors: (1) my empathy and understanding about the difficulty of using a translator, and (2) her comfort in talking with me from the outset. I did not want her to speak with yet another professional, even less someone who might not be able to speak her native language.

We met at noon twice a week, and I also met with Allyson twice a week after she got out of preschool on the days her mother came to see me.

Stephanie was a remarkable young woman. From the time she was very young, she dreamed of coming to the States and getting an education. She had been influenced by an aunt who had traveled to New York early in her life and become a successful businessperson in the field of computers. She admired the fact that her aunt had become a U.S. citizen and had made something of her life. She added that this aunt was quite different from her mother, who was less sophisticated, couldn't read or drive, and was content being a mother to her five children. "My mother is a sad story," she said, "always a martyr, always giving up her life for others." Stephanie insisted that she would not follow in her mother's footsteps and would instead learn something that she could do that would give her financial freedom. Stephanie revealed that someday she wanted to go to community college and study nursing—she commented on how wonderful the nurse had been who supervised her rape exam.

Stephanie cried a lot about her boyfriend, Allyson's father, Diego. She described their courtship, how he had been her first (and last) sexual relationship, and how betrayed she felt when he left her. She bemoaned having "given away her virginity" and hoped her daughter would have sex only when married. She also regretted trusting him enough to allow him to live with her for the year they had been together. She noted that she was completely "duped" by him and would never let anyone trick her again. The first time I ever saw her smile was when she said that the next man who wanted her would have to "put a ring on it!" pointing to her left hand.

We approached the subject of the rape cautiously, building a foundational therapy relationship first. Stephanie stated that she knew that she would have to talk about it at some point to get it out of her head. She complained that it was "taking over" too much of her life: she was having flashbacks, cried without provocation, froze up around certain people, and was irritable and angry, mostly at her parents but sometimes at Allyson too. Stephanie identified her lack of energy, maybe depression, as what she hated the most and wanted to feel motivated to do something constructive with her life, as she had been in her past. She asked specifically what it would take to keep all these ugly memories out of her head, and I described a therapeutic process in which she would externalize her thoughts and feelings so that she could process the impact of the trauma and lessen its impact on her life. I went over what would be considered "trauma processing" and told her that it may not have immediate outcomes but over time would likely help her feel more in control. When I told her that the goal would be for her to be able to speak about what happened to her without feeling overwhelmed and setting aside feelings of guilt and shame that most victims feel, she noted that she was ready to start and would do whatever it took. Of course, her resolve was tested many times; sometimes she felt it was too painful to remember details and to describe them to me. I gave her the options of drawing, using miniatures, making sand pictures, and journaling. She wrote amazing poems, and with her permission, I have translated one of her most powerful missives:

> I will keep fighting you as long as it takes
> I will not look away
> I will not stay down
> I will stand and speak and point to your ugliness
> I will think of you in jail
> And know that I fought back
> Keeping others safe from you
> Now and forever
> I am patient, I am bold, I stand tall

We did trauma work as described by Foa and colleagues (Foa & Rothbaum, 1998), and she was able to capture the events in real time, releasing her anguish, expressing her rage, and managing her painful memories. As we did this work, her symptoms diminished and her motivation returned. Her attention also turned back to her daughter. As they resumed familiar activities, shared warmth and affection, and renewed feelings of safety and security, Allyson's symptoms also decreased, to the delight of her teacher and extended family.

Allyson had progressed well in treatment. The final step was for Stephanie and Allyson, fortified by their individual work, to come together and share what they had accomplished.

PARALLEL TRAUMA-FOCUSED TREATMENT OF MOTHER AND DAUGHTER

I told both Allyson and Stephanie that we were going to have some time together in the same room, at the same time, so that Allyson and Stephanie could take a look at this very difficult event that they experienced together. The hope was that, by taking a look at what had happened together, they would feel stronger (and possibly closer). At this point, my goal was to help mother and daughter co-create and share with each other their narrative in a way that was age-appropriate for Allyson and emphasized mastery and survival for them both. I had coached Stephanie about creating a safe and supportive environment with unconditional acceptance of Allyson's play and behavior. I encouraged her to look for, and punctuate, any thoughts, feelings, or behaviors that were consistent with Allyson's mastery of her traumatic experience. I had two specific objectives when conducting these conjoint sessions: (1) to give Stephanie and Allyson a chance to show and share their individually created narratives to each other, so that the traumatic assault could be stripped of its intensity and be mutually acknowledged, and (2) for Allyson to change her perception of Stephanie as incapable of protecting herself and Allyson in the future. One of the desired outcomes of treatment with children who have witnessed domestic violence is to restore the parent to a status of capable and nurturing protector (Lieberman & van Horn, 2004b). By helping children reestablish their perception of parents as strong and capable, children can begin to anchor their own sense of safety and security.

CONJOINT SESSIONS

The conjoint work began about 6 months after I began to work with both parent and child individually. Stephanie was feeling much better, had done the rigorous work of trauma processing, and had managed to create a cohesive narrative in which she was able to recall most of the traumatic event, except the parts when she was mercifully spared by her dissociative episodes and when she passed out. She had also managed to tell her parents what had happened. She had prepared herself for their criticism and rejection, but Stephanie's mother confided that she herself had also been raped as a teen and had never spoken about it to anyone. Sharing this intimate information gave Stephanie and her mother an opportunity for closeness and mutual empathy, even though it proved fleeting. Since all three females had experienced this traumatic event, I felt it would be useful for the three of them to have a few sessions together if Stephanie and her mother were willing. Stephanie's mother declined to come into therapy but agreed to have conversations with her daughter at home.

Stephanie made great strides in reaching out to friends and in returning to her church activities. She broke her own sense of isolation and stigmatization and eventually said that she was beginning to feel like "her old self." It was at the point when she had strengthened her self-image and had begun to feel increasingly competent that I asked her to participate in this conjoint work.

Allyson had also done individual work on the rape she had witnessed and through posttraumatic play had managed to re-create the story of what she remembered. When I approached her about meeting with her mother, she seemed excited to have her mother join her and to show her around the play therapy office. The first session with Stephanie and Allyson was completely nondirective, with Allyson showing her mom everything in the room, even some things she had never played with herself.

In the second session, I told Allyson that she could have some time to do "whatever she wanted" with her mom but that before she did that, her mom had something that she wanted to talk to her about. Stephanie was a little nervous but ready to have this dialogue with her daughter. She started out by saying the following: "I know that you remember when that man came into our house and hurt me." Allyson looked at her mom and became still. "We've never talked about it because I was hoping that we would both forget what happened. But now I know that it's very hard to forget about it because it was so scary and I was so hurt that I couldn't help you or hold you."

Allyson rushed to the sand tray miniatures and grabbed the "mean man," bringing it back to her mother. "This is the mean man, Mami. He's the one that hurt you. He's mean." "Yes," her mother said, "he was mean and he hurt me a lot and now he's in jail being punished." Allyson asked, "Why did he hurt you, Mami?" and Stephanie said softly, "I don't know mija; some people do not have God in their hearts and they are mean." Allyson kept talking, seemingly wanting to get in everything she had wanted to say. "I kept coming to your room, Mami, but I was scared and running away." Stephanie said, "You are a little girl, not a grown-up, there was nothing you could do. You are a brave and sweet girl, and there was nothing you could do to help me because the man was strong and bigger than us." "I hate him," Allyson said, throwing the miniature of the mean man on the floor.

This dialogue served as the foundation for five sessions in which Stephanie and Allyson told each other the stories they remembered. The following highlights occurred during this time.

Second Session

Allyson feigned illness and asked to be held in her mother's arms throughout most of the session. I encouraged Stephanie to simply hold and rock her daughter, and Stephanie spontaneously began to sing a lullaby. While she did this, Allyson began to twirl her mother's hair around her finger and Stephanie allowed her to do so. I put soft music in the background, and mother sang slowly in her child's ear. The refrain was "ah, ah, ah . . . ah, ah, ah." Allyson's face was relaxed and content, and toward the end of the session she grabbed a little doll from the doll's crib and brought it over to her mother. "This is *my* baby," she said, and she rocked her and sang the lullaby she had learned from her mother. They sat together, rocking and humming until the end of the session, and it seemed to me that this might have been Allyson's way of getting her needs met by her mother and ensuring that her mother would be available for nurturing in the play therapy session.

Third Session

This session was quite different: Allyson pushed the door open and went into the play therapy office, with her mother and myself following behind. I noticed immediately that Allyson had placed familiar objects in the tray. The objects signaled her willingness to "show" her mother about the rape and how she had experienced it. Allyson had done some difficult work with these objects. She had externalized the event of the rape, as well as showing behaviors that occurred while her mother was unable to move. These included one particular behavior that seemed compelling and powerful to Allyson: coming in and out of her room to check on her mother. Allyson placed a baby in the sand tray and put a little fence around it, stating that it was "the baby's room." She then opened and closed one of the fences to indicate that the child could come out at will. "Where is the baby going?" I asked Allyson, and she answered, "You know." I respected her ambivalence about playing out this difficult scenario with her mother in the room, and she did not respond further. She then looked up and asked her mother to go sit in the adjacent room. Stephanie agreed to do so, and then Allyson came in and out, in and out of the room, saying hi to her mother, sitting on her lap, asking her mom to cover up her eyes and guess where she was standing in the room, and throwing a small pillow back and forth between the rooms. Stephanie would find the pillow, pick it up, and throw it back into Allyson's room. This seemed like purposeful play that made way for the narrative that followed the next session.

Fourth Session

Allyson brought her mom into the play therapy office and asked her to sit next to the sand tray. "I'm going to show you my story," she said. Stephanie sat and listened attentively. "This is about the day the bad man hurt you." She proceeded to grab the baby and mother miniature that she had used during individual therapy, as well as the figure she called "the bad man." "Mommy," she said, "I remember that you were crying, and I heard you and came to see you; do you remember?" "Yes," Stephanie said, "that was a terrible time, but I remember seeing you." "You told me to go away." "Yes," Stephanie said, putting her hand around her daughter's waist, "I wanted to make sure you would be safe." "I was scared, Mommy," Allyson said and folded into her mother's arms. "I know you were scared, baby, so was I." They now spoke in Spanish, and Allyson told her what she had seen, how scared she had been, and how she didn't know what to do. She was "the most scared" when her mom seemed to fall asleep and couldn't see her and when she saw blood under her mom's head. She then told her that she went to get help for her next door, even though she was "really, really scared to go." Stephanie told Allyson how proud she was of her and how brave she had been; Stephanie also told her that she would not have gotten the help she needed without her. Allyson had tears in her eyes when she asked, "You're not mad at me?" Stephanie seemed horrified at the thought and told Allyson that she was only mad at the bad man who had hurt her but not at her." They hugged for a long time.

Fifth Session

This session concluded this phase of therapy and consisted of Stephanie telling Allyson her story and what had happened. Stephanie did a great job talking about her feelings during and after the scary event and talked about all the things she had done afterward to make sure the bad man did not hurt anyone else. Allyson told her mom that she was brave too, just like her. They were able to ask questions of each other and share similar feelings during and after the event. This coauthoring of a more ample joint narrative seemed to solidify their relationship, create opportunities for clarification, and provide a way for Allyson to think of her mother as a brave and competent person who could keep her safe in the future.

Stephanie told me that little conversation occurred once the sessions were over and that Allyson seemed to need and want physical comforting much more than before. Stephanie said she came to realize that she found comfort in her child's arms as well, which made her realize that she needed to reach out to her own mother. About 2 months later, we met to discuss how Allyson and Stephanie could show their mother/grandmother what they had endured. Stephanie called me after she met with her mother to tell me it had gone well.

Stephanie expressed her gratitude to me time and time again. She thanked me for the guidance and for giving her the words to help her child. I shared my admiration of her and her willingness to do painful work, motivated by her desire to be a better parent to her child. I especially pointed out her courage and willingness to face and address her fears. For the most part, she felt that she had adequately worked on the trauma she had endured, but every now and then some external event would trigger the event and interrupt her normal functioning. Allyson responded positively to therapy, and her behavior outside the sessions began to improve and return to her pre-rape functioning. Her teachers noticed improved behavior and a return to her prior positive outlook.

CONCLUSION

Witnessing loved ones undergo traumatic events can leave children traumatized themselves. Allyson witnessed her mother's rape by a stranger that lasted a number of hours. As a result, the child felt helpless and acutely frightened. Allyson coped as well as she could under these horrific circumstances but her behavioral adjustment suffered. Allyson's behavioral problems signaled her distress, and therapy was required to help her deal with the traumatic impact she was experiencing. In individual therapy, Allyson was able to identify and access posttraumatic play that allowed her to externalize her worries and concerns. In conjoint sessions, having the mother witness her play further empowered Allyson and allowed the mother–child dyad to face the trauma together and regain a sense of power and control by re-creating the situation and giving voice to their fears and pain. This conjoint treatment was also critical to enhancing attachment between Allyson and her mother, which had been compromised by the sexual assault that rendered mother helpless in her daughter's eyes. Stephanie's role as a protector of her daughter's safety had been gravely damaged, and in order to move forward, Allyson's feelings and needs had to take center stage, in a way they had not when Stephanie was debilitated by her attacker. The last 15 minutes of each of these conjoint sessions included the mother holding and rocking her daughter, singing to her and comforting her, declaring that nothing like that would ever happen again.

Appendix

Checklist for Posttraumatic Play

Child's Name _____ Date of Session _____ Session No. _____

Dynamic Posttraumatic Play

- ☐ Affect variable
- ☐ Seeks interactions with clinician
- ☐ Available for emotional connection
- ☐ Breath fluid
- ☐ Physical movement is fluid
- ☐ Evidence of release
- ☐ Focused investment in play
- ☐ Story starts/ends differently
- ☐ Story has new information/ characters
- ☐ Presence of new themes
- ☐ Play occurs in different locations in room
- ☐ Adaptive outcomes emerge
- ☐ Rigidity loosens over time
- ☐ New characters are added/deleted
- ☐ Role playing emerges
- ☐ Child's voice is given to story characters
- ☐ Temporary increase of symptoms
- ☐ At-home behavior improves

Toxic Posttraumatic Play

- ☐ Affect constricted/flat
- ☐ Play is focused and isolated
- ☐ Unavailable for emotional connect
- ☐ Breath shallow/holds breath
- ☐ Physical tension
- ☐ No evidence of release
- ☐ Rigid interaction with play
- ☐ Story starts/ends unvaried
- ☐ Story is repetitive, without change
- ☐ Thematic material remains fixed
- ☐ Play must be presented in the same place
- ☐ No new outcomes emerge
- ☐ Play remains rigid
- ☐ No new characters are introduced
- ☐ Play still: No role playing (maybe play stagnant?)
- ☐ Child's voice is not present
- ☐ Symptoms increase and stabilize
- ☐ At-home behavior deteriorates

References

Badenoch, B. (2008). *Being a brain-wise therapist: A practical guide to interpersonal neurobiology.* New York: Norton.

Blaustein, M. E., & Kinniburgh, K. M. (2010). *Treating traumatic stress in children and adolescents: How to foster resilience through attachment, self-regulation, and competency.* New York: Guilford Press.

Booth, P. B., & Jernberg, A. M. (2009). *Theraplay: Helping parents and children build better relationships through attachment-based play.* New York: Wiley.

Bratton, S., Landreth, G. L., Kellam, T., & Blackard, S. R. (2006). *Child–parent relationship therapy (CPRT) treatment manual: A 10-session filial therapy model for training parents.* New York: Routledge.

Bratton, S. C., Ray, D., Rhine, T., & Jones, L. (2005). The efficacy of play therapy with children: A meta-analytic review of treatment outcomes. *Professional Psychology: Research and Practice, 36*(4), 376–390.

Briere, J., & Scott, C. (2006). *Principles of trauma therapy: A guide to symptoms, evaluation, and treatment.* Thousand Oaks, CA: Sage.

Chapman, L. (2014a). *Neurobiologically informed trauma therapy with children and adolescents: Understanding mechanisms of change.* New York: Norton.

Chapman, L. (2014b). Treating acute traumatic episodes: A brief intervention for integration. In *Neurobiologically informed trauma therapy with children and adolescents: Understanding mechanisms of change* (pp. 19–49). New York: Norton.

Cohen, E. (2009). Parenting in the throes of traumatic events: Risks and protection. In D. Brown, R. Pat-Horenczyk, & J. D. Ford (Eds.), *Treating traumatized children: Risk, resilience and recovery* (pp. 72–84). New York: Routledge.

Cohen, E., Chazan, S., Lerner, M., & Maimon, E. (2010). Posttraumatic play in young children exposed to terrorism: An empirical study. *Infant Mental Health Journal, 31*(2), 159–181.

Cohen, J. A., & Mannarino, A. P. (1998). Interventions for sexually abused children: Initial treatment outcome findings. *Child Maltreatment, 3,* 17–26.

Cohen, J. A., & Mannarino, A. P. (2008). Trauma-focused cognitive behavioral therapy for children and parents. *Child and Adolescent Mental Health, 13*(4), 158–162.

Cohen, J. A., Mannarino, A. P., & Deblinger, E. (2006). *Treating trauma and traumatic grief in children and adolescents.* New York: Guilford Press.

Dripchak, V. L. (2007). Posttraumatic play: Towards acceptance and resolution. *Journal of Clinical Social Work, 35,* 125–134.

Erikson, E. H. (1950). *Childhood and society.* New York: Norton.

Eth, S., & Pynoos, R. S. (1984). Developmental perspectives on psychic trauma in children. In C. E. Figley (Ed.), *Trauma and its wake* (pp. 36–52). New York: Brunner/Mazel.

Eth, S., & Pynoos, R. S. (1985). Interaction of trauma and grief in childhood. In S. Eth & R. S. Pynoos (Eds.), *Post-traumatic stress disorder in children* (pp. 169–186). Washington, DC: American Psychiatric Press.

Eyberg, S. M. (1988). Parent–child interaction therapy: Integration of traditional and behavioral concerns. *Child and Family Behavior Therapy, 10*(1), 33–46.

Fenichel, E. (Ed.). (1994). Collected works. *Zero to Three/National Center for Clinical Infant Programs, 14*(6), 1–50.

Findling, J. H., Bratton, S. C., & Henson, R. K. (2006). Development of the Trauma Play Scale: An observation-based assessment of the impact of trauma on the play therapy behaviors of young children. *International Journal of Play Therapy, 15*(1), 7–36.

Foa, E. B., & Rothbaum, B. O. (1998). *Treating the trauma of rape: Cognitive-behavioral therapy for PTSD.* New York: Guilford Press

Ford, J. D., & Courtois, C. A. (Eds.). (2013). *Treating complex stress disorders in children and adolescents: Scientific foundations and therapeutic models.* New York: Guilford Press.

Freud, S. (1958). Remembering, repeating, and working through. In J. Strachey (Ed. and Trans.), *The standard edition of the complete psychological work of Sigmund Freud* (Vol. 12, pp. 147–156). London: Hogarth Press. (Original work published 1914)

Gibbs, M. S. (1989). Factors in the victim that mediate between disaster and psychopathology: A review. *Journal of Traumatic Stress, 2,* 489–514.

Gil, E. (1998). Understanding and responding to post-trauma play. *Play Therapy Association Newsletter, 17*(1), 7–10.

Gil, E. (2006a). Scotty, the castle, and the princess guard. In *Helping abused and traumatized children: Integrating directive and nondirective approaches* (pp. 175–191). New York: Guilford Press.

Gil, E. (2006b). *Helping abused and traumatized children: Integrating directive and nondirective approaches.* New York: Guilford Press.

Gil, E. (2006c). *Play therapy for severe psychological trauma* [DVD]. New York: Guilford Press.

Gil, E. (2012). Trauma-focused integrated play therapy. In P. Goodyear-Brown (Ed.), *Handbook of child sexual abuse: Identification, assessment, and treatment* (pp. 251–278). New York: Wiley.

Gil, E. (Ed.). (2013). *Working with children to heal interspersonal trauma: The power of play.* New York: Guilford Press.

Gil, E. (2015a). Reunifying families after critical separations: An integrative play therapy approach to building and strengthening family ties. In D. A. Crenshaw & A. L. Stewart (Eds.), *Play therapy: A comprehensive guide to theory and practice* (pp. 353–369). New York: Guilford Press.

Gil, E. (2015b). Posttraumatic play: A robust path to resilience. In D. A. Crenshaw, R. Brooks, & S. Goldstein (Eds.), *Play therapy interventions to enhance resilience* (pp. 107–125). New York: Guilford Press.

Gil, E. (2015c). *Play in family therapy* (2nd ed.). New York: Guilford Press.

Gil, E., & Pfeifer, L. (2016). Issues of culture and diversity in play therapy. In K. J. O'Connor, C. E. Schaefer, & L. D. Braverman (Eds.), *Handbook of play therapy* (2nd ed., pp. 599–612). New York: Wiley.

Goodman, R. F., & Fahnestock, A. H. (2002). *The day our world changed: Children's art of 9/11.* New York: Harry N. Abrams.

Guerney, L. (2000). Filial therapy into the 21st century. *International Journal of Play Therapy, 9*(2), 1–17.

Hall, T. M., Kaduson, H. G., & Schaefer, C. E. (2002). Fifteen effective play therapy techniques. *Professional Psychology: Research and Practice, 33*(6), 515–522.

Hopkins, S., Huici, V., & Bermudez, D. (2005). Therapeutic play with Hispanic clients. In E. Gil & A. A. Drewes (Eds.), *Cultural issues in play therapy* (pp. 148–167). New York: Guilford Press.

Jung, C. G. (1928). *Contributions to analytical psychology.* New York: Harcourt, Brace.

Kilpatrick, K. L., & Williams, L. M. (1998). Potential mediators of posttraumatic stress disorder in child witnesses to domestic violence. *Child Abuse and Neglect, 22*(4), 319–330.

Lanktree, C. B., & Briere, J. N. (2017). *Treating complex trauma in children and their families: An integrative approach.* Thousand Oaks, CA: Sage.

Levine, P., & van der Kolk, B. (2015). *Trauma and memory: Brain and body in a search for the living past: A practical guide for understanding and working with traumatic memory.* Berkeley, CA: North Atlantic Press.

Levy, D. (1938). Release therapy in young children. *Psychiatry, 1,* 387–390.

Lieberman, A. F., & van Horn, P. (2004a). Assessment and treatment of young children exposed to traumatic events. In J. D. Osofsky (Ed.), *Young children and trauma* (pp. 111–138). New York: Guilford Press.

Lieberman, A. F., & van Horn, P. (2004b). *Don't hit my mommy!: A manual for child–parent psychotherapy with young witnesses of family violence.* Washington, DC: Zero to Three.

Malchiodi, C. A. (Ed.). (2003). *Handbook of art therapy.* New York: Guilford Press.

Malchiodi, C. A. (2012, March 6). Trauma-informed expressive art therapy. *Psychology Today* blog.

Marans, S., Mayes, L. C., & Colonna, A. B. (1993). Psychoanalytic views of children's play. In A. J. Solnit, D. J. Cohen, & P. B. Neubauer (Eds.), *The many meanings of play: A psychoanalytic perspective* (pp. 9–28). New Haven, CT: Yale University Press.

Marvasti, J. A. (1994). Please hurt me again: Posttraumatic play therapy with an abused child. In T. Kottman & C. Schaefer (Eds.), *Play therapy in action: A casebook for practitioners* (pp. 485–525). Lanham, MD: Jason Aronson.

Mills, J. (2007). *Butterfly wisdom, four passages to transformation.* Phoenix, AZ: Imaginal Press.

Nader, K., & Pynoos, R. S. (1991). Play and drawing techniques as tools for interviewing traumatized children. In C. E. Schaefer, K. Gitlin, & A. Sandgrun (Eds.), *Play diagnosis and assessment* (pp. 375–389). New York: Wiley.

Perry, B. D. (2001). The neurodevelopmental impact of violence in childhood. In D. Schetky & E. Benedek (Eds.), *Textbook of child and adolescent forensic psychiatry* (pp. 221–238). Washington, DC: American Psychiatric Press.

Perry, B. D., & Dobson, C. L. (2013). The neurosequential nodel of therapeutics. In J. D. Ford & C. A. Courtois (Eds.), *Treating complex traumatic stress disorders in children and adolescents* (pp. 249–260). New York: Guilford Press.

Perry, B. D., & Szalavitz, M. (2006). *The boy who was raised as a dog: And other stories from a child psychiatrist's notebook—What traumatized children can teach us about loss, love, and healing.* New York: Basic Books.

Powell, B., Cooper, G., Hoffman, K., & Marvin, B. (2013). *The circle of security intervention: Enhancing attachment in early parent–child relationships.* New York: Guilford Press.

Pynoos, R. S., & Eth, S. (1985). Introduction: Post-traumatic stress disorders in childhood: A new perspective. In S. Eth & R. S. Pynoos (Eds.), *Post-traumatic stress disorder in children* (pp. xi–xvi). Washington, DC: American Psychiatric Press.

Pynoos, R. S., & Eth, S. (1986). Witness to violence: The child interview. *Journal of the American Academy of Child Psychiatry, 25,* 306–319.

Pynoos, R. S., & Nader, K. (1989). Case study *"Sniper."* In R. Spitzer, M. Gibbon, A. Skodol, J. B. W. Williams, & M. B. First (Eds.), *Case book: DSM-III-R.* Washington, DC: American Psychiatric Press.

Pynoos, R. S., & Nader, K. (1990). Mental health disturbances in children exposed to disaster: Prevention intervention strategies. In S. Goldston, J. Yager, C. M. Heinicke, & R. S. Pynoos (Eds.), *Preventing mental health disturbances in childhood* (pp. 211–234). Washington, DC: American Psychiatric Press.

Pynoos, R. S., & Nader, K. (1993). Issues in the treatment of posttraumatic stress disorder in children and adolescents. In J. Wilson & B. Raphael (Eds.), *International handbook of traumatic stress syndromes* (pp. 535–549). New York: Plenum Press.

Pynoos, R. S., Nader, K., & March, J. (1991). Childhood post-traumatic stress. In J. Weiner (Ed.), *Textbook of child and adolescent psychiatry* (pp. 955–961). Washington, DC: American Psychiatric Press.

Salmon, K., & Bryant, R. A. (2002). Posttraumatic stress disorder in children: The influence of developmental factors. *Clinical Psychology Review, 22,* 163–188.

Sandved, K. B. (1996). *Butterfly alphabet.* New York: Scholastic.

Saylor, C. F., Swenson, C. C., & Powell, P. (1992). Hurricane Hugo blows down the broccoli: Preschoolers post-disaster play and adjustment. *Child Psychiatry and Human Development, 22,* 139–149.

Saunders, B. E., Berliner, L., & Hanson, R. F. (Eds.). (2003, January 15). *Child physical and sexual abuse: Guidelines for treatment.* Charleston, SC: National Crime Victims Research and Treatment Center.

Saywitz, K. J., Mannarino, A. P., Berliner, L. & Cohen, J. A. (2000). Treatment for sexually abused children and adolescents. *American Psychologist, 55*(9), 1040–1049.

Schaefer, C. E. (1994). Play therapy for psychic trauma in children. In K. J. O'Connor & C. E. Schaefer (Eds.), *Handbook of play therapy: Vol 2. Advances and innovations* (pp. 297–318). New York: Wiley.

Schaefer, C. E., & Carey, L. (1994). *Family play therapy.* New York: Jason Aronson.

Schaefer, C. E., & Drewes, A. A. (Eds.). (2010). *School-based play therapy* (2nd ed.). Hoboken, NJ: Wiley.

Schaefer, C. E., & Drewes, A. A. (2013). *The therapeutic powers of play: 20 core agents of change* (2nd ed.). Hoboken, NJ: Wiley .

Shelby, J. (1997). Rubble, disruption, and tears: Helping young survivors of natural disaster. In H. Kaduson, D. M. Cangelosi, & C. E. Schaefer (Eds.), *The playing cure* (pp. 143–169). Northvale, NJ: Jason Aronson.

Shelby, J. (1999, November). *Crisis intervention with children following Hurricane Andrew.* Poster session presented at the annual meeting of the International Society for Traumatic Stress Studies, Miami, FL.

Shelby, J., & Felix, E. D. (2005). Posttraumatic play therapy: The need for an integrated model of directive and nondirective approaches. In L. A. Reddy, T. M. Files-Hall, & C. E. Schaefer (Eds.), *Empirically based play interventions for children* (pp. 79–103). Washington, DC: American Psychological Association.

Siegel, D. J., & Bryson, T. P. (2011). *The whole-brain child: 12 revolutionary strategies to nurture your child's developing mind, survive everyday parenting struggles, and help your family thrive.* New York: Delacorte Press.

Silberg, J. L. (2012). *The child survivor: Healing developmental trauma and dissociation.* New York: Routledge.

Silverman, W. K., & La Greca, A. M. (2002). Children experiencing disasters: Definitions, reactions, and predictors of outcomes. In A. M. La Greca, W. K. Silverman, E. M. Vernberg, & M. C. Roberts (Eds.), *Helping children cope with disasters and terrorism* (pp. 11–33). Washington, DC: American Psychological Association.

Solomon, J. C. (1938). Active play therapy. *American Journal of Orthopsychiatry, 8,* 479–498.

Stover, C. S., & Berkowitz, S. (2005). Assessing violence exposure and trauma symptoms in young children: A critical review of measures, *Journal of Traumatic Stress, 18*(6), 707–717.

Terr, L. (1981). "Forbidden games": Post-traumatic child's play. *American Academy of Child Psychiatry, 20,* 741–760.

Terr, L. (1991). Childhood traumas: An outline and overview. *American Journal of Psychiatry, 148*(1), 10–20.

Terr, L. (1992). *Too scared to cry: Psychic trauma in childhood.* New York: Basic Books.

Thabet, A. A., Karim, K., & Vostanis, P. (2006). Trauma exposure in pre-school children in a war zone. *British Journal of Psychiatry, 188,* 154–158.

Tinnin, L., & Gantt, L. (2013). *The instinctual trauma response: Dual-brain dynamics: A guide for trauma therapy.* Morgantown, WV: Gargoyle Press.

van der Kolk, B. (1989). The compulsion to repeat the trauma. *Psychiatric Clinics of North America, 12*(2), 389–411.

van der Kolk, B. (2005). Developmental trauma disorder: Towards a rational diagnosis for chronically traumatized children. *Psychiatric Annals, 35*(5), 401–408.

van der Kolk, B. (2014). *The body keeps the score: Brain, mind, and body in the healing of trauma.* New York: Viking.

VanFleet, R. (2013). *Filial therapy: Strengthening parent–child relationships through play* (3rd ed.). Sarasota, FL: Professional Resource Press.

Vernberg, E. M. (2002). Intervention approaches following disasters. In A. M. La Greca, W. K. Silverman, E. M. Vernberg, & M. C. Roberts (Eds.), *Helping children cope with disasters and terrorism* (pp. 55–72). Washington, DC: American Psychological Association.

Wilson, R., & Lyons, L. (2013). *Anxious kids, anxious parents: Seven ways to stop the worry cycle and raise courageous and independent children.* Deerfield Beach, FL: Health Communications.

Zero to Three. (2005). *Diagnostic classification of mental health and developmental disorders of infancy and early childhood* (DC:0–3R) (rev. ed.). Washington, DC: Author.

Index

Lightning Source UK Ltd.
Milton Keynes UK
UKOW06n1509270117
293046UK00001B/12/P

9 781462 528837